Human Anatomy and Physiology
© Mometrix Media – flashcardsecrets.com/teas
ATI TEAS Science

What is the nucleus of a cell?

Human Anatomy and Physiology
© Mometrix Media – flashcardsecrets.com/teas
ATI TEAS Science

What are the following nuclear parts of a cell: chromosomes, chromatin, and nucleolus?

Human Anatomy and Physiology
© Mometrix Media – flashcardsecrets.com/teas
ATI TEAS Science

What are the following nuclear parts of a cell: nuclear envelope, nuclear pores, and nucleoplasm?

Human Anatomy and Physiology
© Mometrix Media – flashcardsecrets.com/teas
ATI TEAS Science

Define *cell membrane,* and name the purpose of the cell membrane.

Human Anatomy and Physiology
© Mometrix Media – flashcardsecrets.com/teas
ATI TEAS Science

What are the layers of the cell membrane?

Human Anatomy and Physiology
© Mometrix Media – flashcardsecrets.com/teas
ATI TEAS Science

What are the roles of cholesterol, glycolipids, and proteins in the cell membrane?

Chromosomes: These are highly condensed, threadlike rods of **DNA**. Short for **deoxyribonucleic acid**, DNA is the genetic material that *stores information about the plant or animal.*

Chromatin: This consists of the DNA and protein that make up **chromosomes**.

Nucleolus: This structure contained within the nucleus consists of protein. It is small, round, does not have a membrane, is involved in **protein synthesis**, and synthesizes and stores **RNA (ribonucleic acid)**.

Nucleus (pl. nuclei): This is a small structure that contains the **chromosomes** and regulates the **DNA** of a cell. The nucleus is the defining structure of **eukaryotic cells**, and all eukaryotic cells have a nucleus. The nucleus is responsible for the passing on of genetic traits between generations. The nucleus contains a *nuclear envelope, nucleoplasm, a nucleolus, nuclear pores, chromatin, and ribosomes.*

The **cell membrane**, also referred to as the **plasma membrane**, is a thin semipermeable membrane of lipids and proteins.

The cell membrane isolates the cell from its external environment while still enabling the cell to communicate with that outside environment.

Nuclear envelope: This encloses the structures of the nucleus. It consists of inner and outer membranes made of **lipids**.

Nuclear pores: These are involved in the exchange of material between the nucleus and the **cytoplasm**.

Nucleoplasm: This is the liquid within the nucleus, and is similar to cytoplasm.

Cholesterol in the cell membrane adds stiffness and flexibility.

Glycolipids help the cell to recognize other cells of the organisms.

The **proteins** in the cell membrane help give the cells shape. Special proteins help the cell communicate with its external environment. Other proteins transport molecules across the cell membrane.

The cell membrane consists of a **phospholipid bilayer**, or double layer, with the **hydrophilic ends** of the outer layer facing the external environment, the inner layer facing the inside of the cell, and the **hydrophobic ends** facing each other.

What sizes of molecules are allowed to pass through a cell membrane?

What types of charges of ions are repelled or attracted to a cell membrane?

What happens to molecules that are not able to diffuse through the cell membrane?

What are the following parts of a cell structure: ribosomes, golgi complex, and vacuoles?

What are the following parts of a cell structure: vesicle, cytoskeleton, and microtubules?

What are the following parts of a cell structure: cytosol, cytoplasm, and cell membrane?

The charge of the **ions** on the cell's surface also either attracts or repels ions. Ions with like charges are repelled, and ions with opposite charges are attracted to the cell's surface.

With regard to molecule size, the cell membrane allows only small molecules to diffuse through it. **Oxygen** and **water** molecules are small and typically can pass through the cell membrane.

Molecules that are soluble in **phospholipids** can usually pass through the cell membrane.

Many molecules are not able to diffuse the cell membrane, and, if needed, those molecules must be moved through by active transport and **vesicles**.

Ribosomes: Ribosomes are involved in *synthesizing proteins from amino acids*. They are numerous, making up about one quarter of the cell. Some cells contain thousands of ribosomes. Some are mobile and some are embedded in the rough **endoplasmic reticulum**.

Golgi complex (Golgi apparatus): This is involved in *synthesizing materials* such as proteins that are transported out of the cell. It is located near the nucleus and consists of layers of **membranes**.

Vacuoles: These are sacs used for *storage, digestion, and waste removal*. There is one large vacuole in plant cells. Animal cells have small, sometimes numerous vacuoles.

Cytosol: This is the *liquid material in the cell*. It is mostly water, but also contains some floating molecules.

Cytoplasm: This is a general term that refers to cytosol and the substructures (organelles) found *within the plasma membrane*, but not within the nucleus.

Cell membrane (plasma membrane): This defines the cell by acting as a *barrier*. It helps keeps cytoplasm in and substances located outside the cell out. It also determines what is allowed to enter and exit the cell.

Vesicle: This is a small organelle within a cell. It has a membrane and performs varying functions, including *moving materials within a cell*.

Cytoskeleton: This consists of **microtubules** that help *shape and support the cell*.

Microtubules: These are part of the **cytoskeleton** and help *support the cell*. They are made of protein.

Name the two types of endoplasmic reticulum, and describe some of the features of the endoplasmic reticulum.

Describe the structure and explain the role of mitochondria.

What are the four main functions of mitochondria?

What are the contents of mitochondria?

Explain the results of chemical reactions that occur between the folds of mitochondria.

What are the following parts of a cell structure: centrosome, centriole, and lysosome?

Mitochondrion (pl. mitochondria): These cell structures vary in terms of size and quantity. Some cells may have one mitochondrion, while others have thousands.

This structure performs various functions such as *generating ATP*, and is also involved in *cell growth and death*. Mitochondria contain their own DNA that is separate from that contained in the nucleus.

Mitochondria consist of an inner and outer membrane. The inner membrane encloses the **matrix**, which contains the **mitochondrial DNA** (mtDNA) and ribosomes. Between the inner and outer membranes are **folds** (cristae).

Centrosome: This is comprised of the pair of **centrioles** located at right angles to each other and surrounded by protein. The centrosome is involved in *mitosis and the cell cycle*.

Centriole: These are cylinder-shaped structures near the nucleus that are involved in *cellular division*. Each cylinder consists of nine groups of three **microtubules**. Centrioles occur in pairs.

Lysosome: This *digests proteins, lipids, and carbohydrates*, and also *transports undigested substances* to the cell membrane so they can be removed. The shape of a lysosome depends on the material being transported.

Endoplasmic reticulum: The two types of endoplasmic reticulum are **rough** (has ribosomes on the surface) and **smooth** (does not have ribosomes on the surface).

It is a tubular network that comprises the *transport system of a cell*. It is fused to the nuclear membrane and extends through the cytoplasm to the cell membrane.

Mitochondria can be involved in many functions, their main one being *supplying the cell with energy*.

The four main functions of mitochondria are: the production of **cell energy**, **cell signaling** (how communications are carried out within a cell, **cellular differentiation** (the process whereby a non-differentiated cell becomes transformed into a cell with a more specialized purpose), and **cell cycle and growth regulation** (the process whereby the cell gets ready to reproduce and reproduces).

Chemical reactions occur here that release energy, control water levels in cells, and recycle and create proteins and fats. **Aerobic respiration** also occurs in the mitochondria.

What are the following parts of a cell structure: cilia and flagella?

What is the cell cycle?

How long does the cell cycle take to complete?

What are mitosis and meiosis?

Define *cell differentiation*, name what controls this process, and give a brief overview of the steps of cell differentiation.

How is gastrulation an example of cell differentiation?

The term **cell cycle** refers to the process by which a cell **reproduces**, which involves *cell growth, the duplication of genetic material, and cell division.*

Complex organisms with many cells use the cell cycle to replace cells as they lose their functionality and wear out.

Cilia (singular: cilium): These are appendages extending from the surface of the cell, the movement of which *causes the cell to move*. They can also result in fluid being moved by the cell.

Flagella: These are tail-like structures on cells that use whip-like movements to *help the cell move*. They are similar to cilia, but are usually longer and not as numerous. A cell usually only has one or a few flagella.

The two ways that cells can reproduce are through meiosis and mitosis.

When cells replicate through **mitosis**, the "daughter cell" is an *exact replica* of the parent cell.

When cells divide through **meiosis**, the daughter cells have *different genetic coding* than the parent cell. Meiosis only happens in specialized reproductive cells called **gametes**.

The entire cell cycle in animal cells can take 24 hours. The time required varies among different cell types.

Human skin cells, for example, are constantly reproducing. Some other cells only divide infrequently. Once neurons are mature, they do not grow or divide.

An example of cell differentiation occurs with **gastrulation**—an early phase in the embryonic development of most animals.

During gastrulation, the cells are organized into three primary germ layers: **ectoderm**, **mesoderm**, and **endoderm**. Then, the cells in these layers differentiate into special tissues and organs. For example, the *nervous system* develops from the ectoderm. The *muscular system* develops from the mesoderm. Much of the *digestive system* develops from the endoderm.

The human body is filled with many different types of cells. The process that helps to determine the cell type for each cell is known as **differentiation**. Another way to say this is when a *less-specialized cell becomes a more-specialized cell*.

This process is controlled by the genes of each cell among a group of cells known as a **zygote**. Following the directions of the genes, a cell builds certain proteins and other pieces that set it apart as a specific type of cell.

Human Anatomy and Physiology

What are the interphase and prophase steps of mitosis?

Human Anatomy and Physiology

What are the metaphase and anaphase steps of mitosis?

Human Anatomy and Physiology

What are the telophase and cytokinesis steps of mitosis?

Human Anatomy and Physiology

What are the events that occur during the first phase of meiosis?

Human Anatomy and Physiology

What are the actions of chromosomes during the first phase of meiosis?

Human Anatomy and Physiology

What are the events that occur during the second cell division of meiosis?

Metaphase: The spindle moves to the center of the cell and chromosome pairs align along the center of the spindle structure.

Anaphase: The pairs of chromosomes, called sisters, begin to pull apart, and may bend. When they are separated, they are called **daughter chromosomes**. Grooves appear in the cell membrane.

Interphase: The cell prepares for division by replicating its genetic and cytoplasmic material. Interphase can be further divided into G_1, S, and G_2.

Prophase: The **chromatin** thickens into chromosomes and the **nuclear membrane** begins to disintegrate. Pairs of **centrioles** move to opposite sides of the cell and spindle fibers begin to form. The **mitotic spindle**, formed from cytoskeleton parts, moves chromosomes around within the cell.

Meiosis has the same phases as mitosis, but they happen twice. In addition, different events occur during some phases of meiosis than mitosis.

The events that occur during the first phase of meiosis are interphase (I), prophase (I), metaphase (I), anaphase (I), telophase (I), and cytokinesis (I).

Telophase: The spindle disintegrates, the nuclear membranes reform, and the chromosomes revert to chromatin. In animal cells, the membrane is pinched. In plant cells, a new cell wall begins to form.

Cytokinesis: This is the physical splitting of the cell (including the cytoplasm) into two cells. Some believe this occurs following telophase. Others say it occurs from anaphase, as the cell begins to furrow, through telophase, when the cell actually splits into two.

Each cell goes through a second cell division, which consists of prophase (II), metaphase (II), anaphase (II), telophase (II), and cytokinesis (II).

The second phase of meiosis is similar to the process of mitosis. Meiosis encourages genetic diversity.

During this first phase of meiosis, *chromosomes cross over, genetic material is exchanged, and tetrads of four chromatids are formed*. The nuclear membrane dissolves. Homologous pairs of chromatids are separated and travel to different poles. At this point, there has been one cell division resulting in two cells.

What is the result of the second phase of meiosis?

Define *tissues,* and name the four broad categories of tissues.

What are the following categories of tissues: epithelial, connective, and cartilage?

What are the following categories of tissues: blood and bone?

What are the following categories of tissues: muscle and nervous?

What are organs?

Tissues are groups of cells that work together to perform a specific function.

Tissues can be grouped into four broad categories: **muscle tissue**, **nerve tissue**, **epithelial tissue**, and **connective tissue**.

The result is *four daughter cells* with different sets of chromosomes. The daughter cells are **haploid**, which means they contain half the genetic material of the parent cell.

Blood – Blood transports oxygen to cells and removes wastes. It also carries hormones and defends against disease.

Bone – Bone is a hard tissue that supports and protects softer tissues and organs. Its marrow produces red blood cells.

Epithelial – Tissue in which cells are joined together tightly. *Skin* tissue is an example.

Connective – Connective tissue may be dense, loose or fatty. It protects and binds body parts. Connective tissues include *bone tissue, cartilage, tendons, ligaments, fat, blood, and lymph.*

Cartilage – Cushions and provides structural support for body parts. It has a jelly-like base and is fibrous.

Organs are groups of tissues that work together to perform specific functions.

Muscle – Muscle tissue helps support and move the body. The three types of muscle tissue are *smooth, cardiac, and skeletal.*

Nervous – Nerve tissue is located in the *brain, spinal cord, and nerves.* Cells called neurons form a network through the body that control responses to changes in the external and internal environment. Some send signals to muscles and glands to trigger responses.

How are the hearts of organisms and the gills in fish examples of complex animals having several organs that are grouped in multiple systems?

What are the 11 major organ systems?

What are the three primary body planes?

What are the following terms of direction: medial and lateral?

What are the following terms of direction: proximal and distal?

What are the following terms of direction: anterior, posterior, superior, and inferior?

In mammals, there are 11 major organ systems: **integumentary system, respiratory system, cardiovascular system, endocrine system, nervous system, immune system, digestive system, excretory system, muscular system, skeletal system**, and **reproductive system**.

Complex animals have several organs that are grouped together in multiple **systems**.

For example, the **heart** is specifically designed to pump blood throughout an organism's body. The heart is composed mostly of muscle tissue in the myocardium, but it also contains connective tissue in the blood and membranes, nervous tissue that controls the heart rate, and epithelial tissue in the membranes.

Gills in fish and lungs in reptiles, birds, and mammals are specifically designed to exchange gases. In birds, crops are designed to store food and gizzards are designed to grind food.

Medial means *nearer to the midline* of the body. In anatomical position, the little finger is medial to the thumb.

Lateral is the opposite of medial. It refers to structures further away from the body's midline, at the sides. In anatomical position, the thumb is lateral to the little finger.

The **transverse (or horizontal) plane** divides the patient's body into imaginary upper (*superior*) and lower (*inferior* or *caudal*) halves.

The **sagittal plane** divides the body, or any body part, vertically into right and left sections. The sagittal plane runs parallel to the midline of the body.

The **coronal (or frontal) plane** divides the body, or any body structure, vertically into front and back (*anterior* and *posterior*) sections. The coronal plane runs vertically through the body at right angles to the midline.

Anterior refers to structures in *front*.

Posterior refers to structures *behind*.

Superior means *above*, or closer to the head.

Inferior means *below*, or closer to the feet.

Proximal refers to structures *closer to the center* of the body. The hip is proximal to the knee.

Distal refers to structures *further away from the center* of the body. The knee is distal to the hip.

What are the following terms of direction: cephalad and caudad?

What is the difference between the upper and the lower respiratory system?

What is an alternative to categorizing the respiratory system?

What is included among the airway of the respiratory system?

What are the contents of the lungs?

What are the features of the respiratory muscles?

The **respiratory system** can be divided into the upper and lower respiratory system.

The **upper respiratory system** includes the nose, nasal cavity, mouth, pharynx, and larynx. The **lower respiratory system** includes the trachea, lungs, and bronchial tree.

Alternatively, the components of the respiratory system can be categorized as part of the airway, the lungs, or the respiratory muscles.

Cephalad and **cephalic** are adverbs meaning towards the *head*. **Cranial** is the adjective, meaning of the *skull*.

Caudad is an adverb meaning towards the *tail* or posterior. **Caudal** is the adjective, meaning of the *hindquarters*.

The **airway** includes the nose, nasal cavity, mouth, pharynx, (throat), larynx (voice box), trachea (windpipe), bronchi, and bronchial network.

The airway is lined with **cilia** that trap microbes and debris and sweep them back toward the mouth.

Alternatively, the components of the respiratory system can be categorized as part of the airway, the lungs, or the respiratory muscles.

The respiratory muscles include the diaphragm and the intercostal muscles.

The **diaphragm** is a dome-shaped muscle that separates the thoracic and abdominal cavities.

The **intercostal muscles** are located between the ribs.

The **lungs** are structures that house the **bronchi** and **bronchial network**, which extend into the lungs and terminate in millions of **alveoli** (air sacs).

The walls of the alveoli are only one cell thick, allowing for the exchange of gases with the blood capillaries that surround them.

The right lung has three lobes. The left lung only has two lobes, leaving room for the heart on the left side of the body.

The lungs are surrounded by a **pleural membrane**, which reduces friction between surfaces when breathing.

Name the main function of the respiratory system, and name where this function occurs.

How is the respiratory system responsible for producing speech, filtering air, and producing coughs?

How is the respiratory system responsible for the sense of smell and maintaining acid-base homeostasis?

What happens during inhalation and exhalation?

Explain how air rushes into the lungs and how air is forced out of the lungs.

What portion of the brain stem controls the breathing process?

The respiratory system is responsible for speech. As air passes through the throat, it moves through the **larynx** (voice box), which vibrates and produces sound, before it enters the **trachea** (windpipe).

The respiratory system also filters air. Air is warmed, moistened, and filtered as it passes through the nasal passages before it reaches the lungs.

The respiratory system is vital in cough production. Foreign particles entering the nasal passages or airways are expelled from the body by the respiratory system.

The main function of the respiratory system is to supply the body with **oxygen** and rid the body of **carbon dioxide**.

This exchange of gases occurs in millions of tiny **alveoli**, which are surrounded by blood capillaries.

During the breathing process, the **diaphragm** and the **intercostal muscles** contract to expand the lungs.

During **inspiration** or inhalation, the diaphragm contracts and moves down, increasing the size of the chest cavity.

During **expiration** or exhalation, the intercostal muscles contract and the ribs are pulled inward, decreasing the size of the chest cavity.

The respiratory system functions in the sense of smell. **Chemoreceptors** that are located in the nasal cavity respond to airborne chemicals.

The respiratory system also helps the body maintain acid-base **homeostasis**. Hyperventilation can increase blood pH during **acidosis** (low pH). Slowing breathing during **alkalosis** (high pH) helps to lower blood pH.

The breathing process is controlled by the portion of the brain stem called the **medulla oblongata**.

The medulla oblongata monitors the level of carbon dioxide in the blood and signals the breathing rate to increase when these levels are too high.

As the volume of the chest cavity increases, the pressure inside the chest cavity decreases. Because the outside air is under a greater amount of pressure than the air inside the lungs, air rushes into the lungs.

When the diaphragm and intercostal muscles relax, the size of the chest cavity decreases, forcing air out of the lungs.

Human Anatomy and Physiology
© Mometrix Media – flashcardsecrets.com/teas
ATI TEAS Science

Name the responsibility of the circulatory system, and name the three main parts of this system.

Human Anatomy and Physiology
© Mometrix Media – flashcardsecrets.com/teas
ATI TEAS Science

Do most animals have an open or closed circulatory system?

Human Anatomy and Physiology
© Mometrix Media – flashcardsecrets.com/teas
ATI TEAS Science

What happens to the rate of blood as it moves from larger tubules through smaller tubules?

Human Anatomy and Physiology
© Mometrix Media – flashcardsecrets.com/teas
ATI TEAS Science

Explain what blood does for the human body, and name the number of quarts of blood in the average adult human.

Human Anatomy and Physiology
© Mometrix Media – flashcardsecrets.com/teas
ATI TEAS Science

Name the main components of blood, and name the role and contents of plasma.

Human Anatomy and Physiology
© Mometrix Media – flashcardsecrets.com/teas
ATI TEAS Science

What are red blood cells?

Circulatory systems can be either **open** or **closed**. Most animals have closed systems, where the *heart and blood vessels are continually connected.*

The **circulatory system** is responsible for the internal transport of substances to and from the cells.

The circulatory system usually consists of the following three parts:
- **Blood** – Blood is composed of water, solutes, and other elements in a fluid connective tissue.
- **Blood Vessels** – Tubules of different sizes that transport blood.
- **Heart** – The heart is a muscular pump providing the pressure necessary to keep blood flowing.

Blood helps maintain a healthy internal environment in animals by *carrying raw materials to cells* and *removing waste products.* It helps stabilize internal pH and hosts various kinds of infection fighters.

An adult human has about five quarts of blood.

As the blood moves through the system from larger tubules through smaller ones, the rate slows down. The flow of blood in the **capillary beds**, the smallest tubules, is quite slow.

Red blood cells transport **oxygen** to cells. Red blood cells form in the bone marrow and can live for about four months. These cells are constantly being replaced by fresh ones, keeping the total number relatively stable.

Blood is composed of **red and white blood cells**, **platelets**, and **plasma**.

Plasma constitutes over half of the blood volume. It is mostly water and serves as a solvent. Plasma contains plasma proteins, ions, glucose, amino acids, hormones, and dissolved gases.

What are white blood cells and platelets?

Name the type of muscle tissue that makes up the heart, and explain the structure of the heart.

Describe briefly how the heart functions by contracting and relaxing.

What role does complex electrical system in humans have in the circulatory system?

What are the two main phases of the cardiac cycle?

How does blood move from the superior and inferior venae cavae to being filled in the right ventricle?

The heart is a muscular pump made of **cardiac muscle tissue**.

It has four chambers; each half contains both an **atrium** and a **ventricle**, and the halves are separated by a valve, known as the AV valve. It is located between the ventricle and the artery leading away from the heart.

Valves keep blood moving in a single direction and prevent any backwash into the chambers.

Cardiac muscles are attached to each other and signals for contractions spread rapidly. A complex electrical system controls the heartbeat as cardiac muscle cells produce and conduct electric signals. These muscles are said to be **self-exciting**, needing no external stimuli.

During the first diastole phase, blood flows through the **superior** and **inferior venae cavae**. Because the heart is relaxed, blood flows passively from the atrium through the open **atrioventricular valve** (tricuspid valve) to the right ventricle.

The **sinoatrial (SA) node**, the cardiac pacemaker located in the wall of the right atrium, generates electrical signals, which are carried by the **Purkinje fibers** to the rest of the atrium, stimulating it to contract and fill the right ventricle with blood.

White blood cells defend the body against **infection** and remove various wastes. The types of white blood cells include lymphocytes, neutrophils, monocytes, eosinophils, and basophils.

Platelets are fragments of stem cells and serve an important function in *blood clotting*.

The heart functions by contracting and relaxing. **Atrial contraction** fills the ventricles and **ventricular contraction** empties them, forcing circulation.

This sequence is called the **cardiac cycle**.

The cardiac cycle consists of **diastole** and **systole** phases, which can be further divided into the first and second phases to describe the events of the right and left sides of the heart. However, these events are simultaneously occurring.

What initiates the first systole phase?

In the time between the tricuspid valve closing and blood filing the left ventricle, what happens during the cardiac cycle?

What happens during the second systole phase?

What are the main types of circulation in the circulatory system?

What happens during the coronary circulation?

What happens during the pulmonary circulation?

The tricuspid valve closes, and the **pulmonary semilunar valve** opens. Blood is pumped out the **pulmonary arteries** to the lungs.

Blood returning from the lungs fills the left atrium as part of the second diastole phase.

The SA node triggers **the mitral valve** to open, and blood fills the left ventricle.

The impulse from the SA node is transmitted to the ventricle through the atrioventricular (AV) node, signaling the right ventricle to contract and initiating the first systole phase.

The **circulatory system** includes coronary circulation, pulmonary circulation, and systemic circulation.

During the second systole phase, the mitral valve closes and the **aortic semilunar valve** opens. The left ventricle contracts, and blood is pumped out of the aorta to the rest of the body.

Pulmonary circulation is the flow of blood between the heart and the lungs. Deoxygenated blood flows from the right ventricle to the lungs through **pulmonary arteries**. Oxygenated blood flows back to the left atrium through the **pulmonary veins**.

Coronary circulation is the flow of blood to the heart tissue. Blood enters the **coronary arteries**, which branch off the aorta, supplying major arteries, which enter the heart with oxygenated blood.

The deoxygenated blood returns to the right atrium through the **cardiac veins**, which empty into the **coronary sinus**.

What happens during the systemic circulation?

What happens during the portal circulation?

Define *blood pressure*, *arterial blood pressure*, *arteries*, and *arterioles*.

What are capillary beds and capillaries?

Define *veins*, and name their responsibility.

Name the main function of the lymphatic system, and name the contents of this system.

Systemic circulation is the flow of blood to the entire body with the exception of coronary circulation and pulmonary circulation. Blood exits the left ventricle through the aorta, which branches into the *carotid arteries, subclavian arteries, common iliac arteries, and the renal artery*. Blood returns to the heart through the *jugular veins, subclavian veins, common iliac veins, and renal veins*, which empty into the **superior** and **inferior venae cavae**.

Included in systemic circulation is **portal circulation**, which is the flow of blood from the digestive system to the liver and then to the heart, and **renal circulation**, which is the flow of blood between the heart and the kidneys.

Blood pressure is the fluid pressure generated by the cardiac cycle.

Arterial blood pressure functions by transporting oxygen-poor blood into the lungs and oxygen-rich blood to the body tissues.

Arteries branch into smaller arterioles which contract and expand based on signals from the body.

Arterioles are where adjustments are made in blood delivery to specific areas based on complex communication from body systems.

Capillary beds are diffusion sites for exchanges between blood and interstitial fluid.

A capillary has the thinnest wall of any blood vessel, consisting of a single layer of **endothelial cells**.

Capillaries merge into venules, which in turn merge with larger diameter tubules called **veins**. Veins transport blood from body tissues back to the heart.

Valves inside the veins facilitate this transport. The walls of veins are thin and contain smooth muscle and also function as blood volume reserves.

The main function of the **lymphatic system** is to *return excess tissue fluid to the bloodstream*.

This system consists of transport vessels and lymphoid organs. The lymph vascular system consists of **lymph capillaries, lymph vessels**, and **lymph ducts**.

What are the major functions of the lymph vascular system?

What is included in the lymphoid organs?

Name the location of lymph nodes, and name what each node contains.

What role does the spleen and the thymus play in the lymphatic system?

Name the location of the spleen, and describe the shape and structure of the spleen.

What are the peritoneal ligaments that support the spleen?

Lymphoid organs include the lymph nodes, spleen, appendix, adenoids, thymus, tonsils, and small patches of tissue in the small intestine.

The major functions of the lymph vascular system are:
- The return of excess fluid to the blood.
- The return of protein from the capillaries.
- The transport of fats from the digestive tract.
- The disposal of debris and cellular waste.

The **spleen** filters blood stores of red blood cells and macrophages. The **thymus** secretes hormones and is the major site of lymphocyte production.

Lymph nodes are located at intervals throughout the lymph vessel system.

Each node contains **lymphocytes** and **plasma cells**.

The following **peritoneal ligaments** support the spleen:
- The **gastrolienal ligament** that connects the stomach to the spleen.
- The **lienorenal ligament** that connects the kidney to the spleen.
- The middle section of the **phrenicocolic ligament** (connects the left colic flexure to the thoracic diaphragm).

The **spleen** is in the upper left of the abdomen. It is located behind the stomach and immediately below the diaphragm.

It is about the size of a thick paperback book and weighs just over half a pound. It is made up of **lymphoid tissue**. The blood vessels are connected to the spleen by **splenic sinuses** (modified capillaries).

Human Anatomy and Physiology
© Mometrix Media – flashcardsecrets.com/teas
ATI TEAS Science

What are the main functions of the spleen?

Human Anatomy and Physiology
© Mometrix Media – flashcardsecrets.com/teas
ATI TEAS Science

Explain the following ways in which the digestive system functions: *movement, secretion, digestion, and absorption.*

Human Anatomy and Physiology
© Mometrix Media – flashcardsecrets.com/teas
ATI TEAS Science

What are the contents of the digestive system?

Human Anatomy and Physiology
© Mometrix Media – flashcardsecrets.com/teas
ATI TEAS Science

What is the role of the mouth in the digestive system?

Human Anatomy and Physiology
© Mometrix Media – flashcardsecrets.com/teas
ATI TEAS Science

What are the three main functions of the stomach?

Human Anatomy and Physiology
© Mometrix Media – flashcardsecrets.com/teas
ATI TEAS Science

Name the responsibility of stomach acidity, and explain the role of smooth muscle contractions in the digestive process.

Most digestive systems function by the following means:
- **Movement** – Movement mixes and passes nutrients through the system and eliminates waste.
- **Secretion** – Enzymes, hormones, and other substances necessary for digestion are secreted into the digestive tract.
- **Digestion** – Includes the chemical breakdown of nutrients into smaller units that enter the internal environment.
- **Absorption** – The passage of nutrients through plasma membranes into the blood or lymph and then to the body.

The main functions of the spleen are to *filter unwanted materials* from the blood (including old red blood cells) and to help *fight infections*.

Digestion begins in the mouth with the chewing and mixing of nutrients with **saliva**.

Salivary glands are stimulated and secrete saliva. Saliva contains **enzymes** that initiate the breakdown of starch in digestion. Once swallowed, the food moves down the **pharynx** into the **esophagus** en route to the stomach.

Only humans and other mammals actually chew their food.

The human digestive system consists of the mouth, pharynx, esophagus, stomach, small and large intestine, rectum, and anus.

Protein digestion begins in the stomach. Stomach acidity helps break down the food and make nutrients available for absorption.

Smooth muscle moves the food by **peristalsis**, contracting and relaxing to move nutrients along. Smooth muscle contractions move nutrients into the small intestine where the **absorption** process begins.

As a flexible, muscular sac, the **stomach** has three main functions:
- Mixing and storing food
- Dissolving and degrading food via secretions
- Controlling passage of food into the small intestine

Describe the liver, and name where it is located in the human body.

Name the four lobes that make up the liver, and name the five ligaments that secure the liver to the diaphragm and abdominal walls.

What is the direction of blood as it enters and exits the liver?

What are the many vital functions in the body for which the liver is responsible?

Explain what happens to nutrients that pass through the liver, and name where most nutrients are absorbed in the digestive process.

What role do enzymes and bile have for digestion in the small intestine?

The **liver** is the largest solid organ of the body. It is also the largest gland. It weighs about three pounds and is located below the diaphragm on the right side of the chest.

The liver is made up of four **lobes**. They are called the *right, left, quadrate, and caudate lobes*.

The liver is secured to the diaphragm and abdominal walls by five **ligaments**. They are called the *falciform* (that forms a membrane-like barrier between the right and left lobes), *coronary, right triangular, left triangular, and round ligaments*.

The liver processes all of the blood that passes through the digestive system.

Nutrient-rich blood is supplied to the liver via the **hepatic portal vein**. The **hepatic artery** supplies oxygen-rich blood. Blood leaves the liver through the **hepatic veins**. The liver's functional units are called **lobules** (made up of layers of liver cells).

Blood enters the lobules through branches of the portal vein and hepatic artery. The blood then flows through small channels called **sinusoids**.

The liver is responsible for performing many vital functions in the body including:
- Production of **bile**
- Production of certain **blood plasma proteins**
- Production of **cholesterol** (and certain proteins needed to carry fats)
- Storage of excess glucose in the form of **glycogen** (that can be converted back to glucose when needed)
- Regulation of **amino acids**
- Processing of **hemoglobin** (to store iron)
- Conversion of ammonia (that is poisonous to the body) to **urea** (a waste product excreted in urine)
- **Purification** of the blood (clears out drugs and other toxins)
- Regulation of **blood clotting**
- Controlling infections by boosting **immune factors** and removing bacteria.

Enzymes from the pancreas, liver, and stomach are transported to the small intestine to aid digestion. These enzymes act on *fats, carbohydrates, nucleic acids, and proteins*.

Bile is a secretion of the liver and is particularly useful in breaking down fats. It is stored in the **gall bladder** between meals.

The nutrients (and drugs) that pass through the liver are converted into forms that are appropriate for the body to use.

In the digestive process, most nutrients are absorbed in the **small intestine**.

Human Anatomy and Physiology
© Mometrix Media – flashcardsecrets.com/teas
ATI TEAS Science

What are the absorptive structures in the small intestine that assist with the digestive system?

Human Anatomy and Physiology
© Mometrix Media – flashcardsecrets.com/teas
ATI TEAS Science

Name the purpose and the location of the large intestine in the human body.

Human Anatomy and Physiology
© Mometrix Media – flashcardsecrets.com/teas
ATI TEAS Science

What is the process of waste matter being expelled from the human body?

Human Anatomy and Physiology
© Mometrix Media – flashcardsecrets.com/teas
ATI TEAS Science

What influences the speed at which waste moves through the large intestine?

Human Anatomy and Physiology
© Mometrix Media – flashcardsecrets.com/teas
ATI TEAS Science

Name the length and location of the pancreas, and describe the shape and structure of the pancreas.

Human Anatomy and Physiology
© Mometrix Media – flashcardsecrets.com/teas
ATI TEAS Science

What is the responsibility of the exocrine tissues and the endocrine tissue in the pancreas?

Also called the **colon**, the large intestine concentrates, mixes, and stores waste material.

A little over a meter in length, the colon ascends on the right side of the abdominal cavity, cuts across transversely to the left side, then descends and attaches to the **rectum**, a short tube for waste disposal.

By the time food reaches the lining of the small intestine, it has been reduced to small molecules.

The lining of the small intestine is covered with **villi**, tiny absorptive structures that greatly increase the surface area for interaction with chyme (the semi-liquid mass of partially digested food).

Epithelial cells at the surface of the villi, called **microvilli**, further increase the ability of the small intestine to serve as the *main absorption organ* of the digestive tract.

The speed at which waste moves through the colon is influenced by the volume of fiber and other undigested material present.

Without adequate bulk in the diet, it takes longer to move waste along, sometimes with negative effects. Lack of bulk in the diet has been linked to a number of disorders.

When the rectal wall is distended by waste material, the nervous system triggers an impulse in the body to expel the waste from the rectum. A muscle **sphincter** at the end of the **anus** is stimulated to facilitate the expelling of waste matter.

The pancreas is made up of exocrine and endocrine tissues.

The **exocrine tissue** secretes digestive enzymes from a series of ducts that collectively form the **main pancreatic duct** (that runs the length of the pancreas). The main pancreatic duct connects to the common bile duct near the duodenum.

The **endocrine tissue** secretes hormones (such as insulin) into the bloodstream.

The **pancreas** is six to ten inches long and located at the back of the abdomen behind the stomach.

It is a long, tapered organ. The wider (right) side is called the **head** and the narrower (left) side is called the **tail**.

The head lies near the **duodenum** (the first part of the small intestine) and the tail ends near the **spleen**. The body of the pancreas lies between the head and the tail.

How does blood reach the pancreas?

How does the pancreas assist in digestion?

How are the enzymes secreted by the pancreas made and converted?

What is the need for the pancreas to secrete sodium bicarbonate?

Name what controls the exocrine function of the pancreas, and name where these exocrine secretions are delivered.

What is the task of the human nervous system and how is this process made possible?

The pancreas assists in the digestion of foods by secreting **enzymes** (to the small intestine) that help to break down many foods, especially fats and proteins.

Blood is supplied to the pancreas from the *splenic artery, gastroduodenal artery, and the superior mesenteric artery*.

The pancreas also secretes large amounts of **sodium bicarbonate** to neutralize the stomach acid that reaches the small intestine.

The precursors to these enzymes (called **zymogens**) are produced by groups of exocrine cells (called **acini**).

They are converted, through a chemical reaction in the gut, to the active enzymes (such as **pancreatic lipase** and **amylase**) once they enter the small intestine.

The human **nervous system** senses, interprets, and issues commands as a response to conditions in the body's environment.

This process is made possible by a very complex communication system organized as a grid of **neurons**.

The **exocrine** functions of the pancreas are controlled by hormones released by the stomach and small intestine (duodenum) when food is present.

The exocrine secretions of the pancreas flow into the main pancreatic duct (**Wirsung's duct**) and are delivered to the duodenum through the pancreatic duct.

How are messages sent across the network of the human nervous system?

What is the task of sensory neurons, motor neurons, and interneurons?

What is the responsibility of the dendrites, the cell body, and the axon in the human nervous system?

Describe the spinal cord, and name the responsibility of the spinal cord.

Describe the location of the frontal and the parietal lobe in the brain, and name the responsibility of each lobe.

Describe the location of the occipital and the temporal lobes in the brain, and name the responsibility of each lobe.

Sensory neurons transmit signals to the **central nervous system** (CNS) from the sensory receptors associated with touch, pain, temperature, hearing, sight, smell, and taste.

Motor neurons transmit signals from the CNS to the rest of the body such as by signaling muscles or glands to respond.

Interneurons transmit signals between neurons; for example, interneurons receive transmitted signals between sensory neurons and motor neurons.

Messages are sent across the plasma membrane of neurons through a process called **action potential**. These messages occur when a neuron is stimulated past a necessary threshold. These stimulations occur in a sequence from the stimulation point of one neuron to its contact with another neuron.

At the point of contact, called a **chemical synapse**, a substance is released that stimulates or inhibits the action of the adjoining cell.

This network fans out across the body and forms the framework for the nervous system. The direction the information flows depends on the specific organizations of nerve circuits and pathways.

The **spinal cord** is encased in the bony structure of the **vertebrae**, which protects and supports it.

Its nervous tissue functions mainly with respect to limb movement and internal organ activity. Major nerve tracts ascend and descend from the spinal cord to the brain.

The **dendrites** receive **impulses** from sensory receptors or interneurons and transmit them toward the cell body.

The **cell body** (soma) contains the nucleus of the neuron.

The **axon** transmits the impulses away from the cell body. The axon is insulated by **oligodendrocytes** and the **myelin sheath** with gaps known as the **nodes of Ranvier**. The axon terminates at the synapse.

The **occipital lobe** is located at the back of the head just above the brain stem. This lobe is responsible for *visual input, processing, and output*; specifically nerves from the eyes enter directly into this lobe.

Finally, the **temporal lobes** are located at the left and right sides of the brain. These lobes are responsible for all *auditory input, processing, and output.*

The **frontal lobe** located in the front of the brain is responsible for a short term and working *memory and information processing* as well as *decision-making, planning, and judgment.*

The **parietal lobe** is located slightly toward the back of the brain and the top of the head and is responsible for *sensory input* as well as *spatial positioning of the body.*

What is the role of the cerebellum?

How was the role of the cerebellum discovered?

Name the location of the brain stem, and name the three parts of the brain stem.

Explain how information is transferred from the body to the brain, and name the three human body functions where the brain stem serves an important role.

Name the location and the parts of the midbrain.

Name the location and the role of the pons and the medulla oblongata.

The role of the cerebellum was discovered by exploring the memory of individuals with damaged cerebellums. These individuals were unable to develop stimulus responses when presented via a classical conditioning technique.

Researchers found that this was also the case for automatic responses. For example, when these individuals where presented with a puff or air into their eyes, they did not blink, which would have been the naturally occurring and automatic response in an individual with no brain damage.

The **cerebellum** plays a role in the processing and storing of *implicit memories*. Specifically, for those memories developed during classical conditioning learning techniques.

Information from the body is sent to the brain through the brain stem, and information from the brain is sent to the body through the brain stem.

The brain stem is an important part of *respiratory, digestive, and circulatory functions*.

The **posterior** area of the brain that is connected to the spinal cord is known as the **brain stem**. The **midbrain**, the **pons**, and the **medulla oblongata** are the three parts of the brain stem.

The **pons** comes between the midbrain and the medulla oblongata. Information is sent across the pons from the cerebrum to the medulla and the cerebellum.

The **medulla oblongata** (or medulla) is beneath the midbrain and the pons. The medulla oblongata is the piece of the brain stem that connects the spinal cord to the brain.

The medulla oblongata has an important role with the autonomous nervous system in the *circulatory and respiratory system*.

The **midbrain** lies above the pons and the medulla oblongata.

The parts of the midbrain include the **tectum**, the **tegmentum**, and the **ventral tegmentum**.

Name the nerves that are responsible for triggering the "fight or flight" response, and name the nerves that control basic body function.

Name the task of the autonomic nervous system (ANS), and explain how that task is accomplished.

Name the two divisions of the ANS, and explain the role of these nervous systems.

What is the responsibility of the somatic nervous system?

What is the task of the efferent and afferent nerves?

What are reflex arcs and reflexes?

The **autonomic nervous system** (ANS) maintains **homeostasis** within the body. In general, the ANS controls the functions of the *internal organs, blood vessels, smooth muscle tissues, and glands.*

This is accomplished through the direction of the **hypothalamus**, which is located above the midbrain. The hypothalamus controls the ANS through the brain stem. With this direction from the hypothalamus, the ANS helps maintain a stable body environment (homeostasis) by regulating numerous factors including heart rate, breathing rate, body temperature, and blood pH.

The **peripheral nervous system** consists of the nerves and ganglia throughout the body and includes **sympathetic nerves** that trigger the "fight or flight" response, and the **parasympathetic nerves** which control basic body function.

The **somatic nervous system** (SNS) controls the five senses and the voluntary movement of skeletal muscle. So, this system has all of the neurons that are connected to sense organs.

The ANS consists of two divisions: the sympathetic nervous system and the parasympathetic nervous system.

The **sympathetic nervous system** controls the body's reaction to extreme, stressful, and emergency situations. For example, the sympathetic nervous system increases the heart rate, signals the adrenal glands to secrete adrenaline, triggers the dilation of the pupils, and slows digestion.

The **parasympathetic nervous system** counteracts the effects of the sympathetic nervous system. For example, the parasympathetic nervous system decreases heart rate, signals the adrenal glands to stop secreting adrenaline, constricts the pupils, and returns the digestion process to normal.

The somatic nervous system also performs involuntary movements which are known as reflex arcs.

A **reflex**, the simplest act of the nervous system, is an automatic response without any conscious thought to a stimulus via the reflex arc.

Efferent (motor) and afferent (sensory) nerves help the somatic nervous system operate the senses and the movement of skeletal muscle.

Efferent nerves bring signals from the central nervous system to the sensory organs and the muscles. **Afferent nerves** bring signals from the sensory organs and the muscles to the central nervous system.

Name the simplest nerve pathway in the human body, and explain the order of events that occur with the classic knee-jerk response.

What are the three properties that all muscles have in common?

Name the type of muscular tissue that is a *voluntary muscle*, and explain its features and responsibility.

Name the two types of muscular tissue that are *involuntary muscles*, and explain their features and location in the human body.

How does the interaction of the skeleton and skeletal muscle help move the body?

What is the composition of skeletal muscles and muscle fibers?

All muscles have these three properties in common:
- **Excitability** – All muscle tissues have an *electric gradient* which can reverse when stimulated.
- **Contraction** – All muscle tissues have the ability to *contract*, or shorten.
- **Elongate** – All muscle tissues share the capacity to *elongate*, or relax.

The **reflex arc** is the simplest nerve pathway, which bypasses the brain and is controlled by the spinal cord.

For example, in the classic knee-jerk response (patellar tendon reflex), the stimulus is the reflex hammer hitting the tendon, and the response is the muscle contracting, which jerks the foot upward.

The stimulus is detected by sensory receptors, and a message is sent along a **sensory** (afferent) neuron to one or more **interneurons** in the spinal cord. The interneuron(s) transmit this message to a **motor** (efferent) neuron, which carries the message to the correct **effector** (muscle).

Smooth muscle tissues are *involuntary* muscles that are found in the walls of internal organs such as the stomach, intestines, and blood vessels. Smooth muscle tissues or **visceral tissue** is nonstriated. Smooth muscle cells are shorter and wider than skeletal muscle fibers. Smooth muscle tissue is also found in sphincters or valves that control various openings throughout the body.

Cardiac muscle tissue is *involuntary* muscle that is found only in the heart. Like skeletal muscle cells, cardiac muscle cells are also striated.

Skeletal muscles are *voluntary* muscles that work in pairs to move various parts of the skeleton.

Skeletal muscles are composed of **muscle fibers** (cells) that are bound together in parallel **bundles**. Skeletal muscles are also known as **striated muscle** due to their striped appearance under a microscope.

Skeletal muscles consist of numerous muscle fibers. Each muscle fiber contains a bundle of **myofibrils**, which are composed of multiple repeating contractile units called **sarcomeres**.

Only skeletal muscle interacts with the skeleton to move the body. When they contract, the muscles transmit **force** to the attached bones. Working together, the muscles and bones act as a system of levers which move around the joints.

A small contraction of a muscle can produce a large movement. A limb can be extended and rotated around a joint due to the way the muscles are arranged.

Explain the two protein microfilaments of myofibrils and their differences, and explain the two types of striations in skeletal muscles and their differences.

How does the sliding filament model explain muscle contraction?

What are the functions of the male reproductive system?

Name the pieces of the external structure of the male reproductive system, and explain the functions of each piece.

Name the pieces of the internal structure of the male reproductive system, and explain the functions of each piece.

Name the hormones associated with the male reproductive system, and name the process that is influenced by each hormone.

When an **action potential** (electrical signal) reaches a muscle fiber, **calcium ions** are released.

According to the sliding filament model of muscle contraction, these calcium ions bind to the myosin and actin, which assists in the binding of the **myosin heads** of the thick filaments to the **actin molecules** of the thin filaments.

Adenosine triphosphate released from glucose provides the energy necessary for the contraction.

Myofibrils contain two protein **microfilaments**: a thick filament and a thin filament. The thick filament is composed of the protein **myosin**. The thin filament is composed of the protein **actin**.

The dark bands (**striations**) in skeletal muscles are formed when thick and thin filaments overlap.

Light bands occur where the thin filament is overlapped. Skeletal muscle attraction occurs when the thin filaments slide over the thick filaments shortening the sarcomere.

The external structure includes the penis, scrotum, and testes.

The **penis**, which contains the **urethra**, can fill with blood and become erect, enabling the deposition of semen and sperm into the female reproductive tract during sexual intercourse. The **scrotum** is a sac of skin and smooth muscle that houses the testes and keeps the testes at the proper temperature for **spermatogenesis**. The **testes**, or testicles, are the male gonads, which produce sperm and testosterone.

The functions of the **male reproductive system** are to produce, maintain, and transfer **sperm** and **semen** into the female reproductive tract and to produce and secrete **male hormones**.

The hormones associated with the male reproductive system include:
- **follicle-stimulating hormone**, which stimulates spermatogenesis
- **luteinizing hormone**, which stimulates testosterone production
- **testosterone**, which is responsible for the male sex characteristics.

The internal structure includes the epididymis, vas deferens, ejaculatory ducts, urethra, seminal vesicles, prostate gland, and bulbourethral glands.

The **epididymis** stores the sperm as it matures. Mature sperm moves from the epididymis through the **vas deferens** to the **ejaculatory duct**. The **seminal vesicles** secrete alkaline fluids with proteins and mucus into the ejaculatory duct, also. The **prostate gland** secretes a milky white fluid with proteins and enzymes as part of the semen. The **bulbourethral**, or Cowper's, glands secrete a fluid into the urethra to neutralize the acidity in the urethra.

What are the functions of the female reproductive system?

Name the pieces of the external portion of the female reproductive system, and explain the functions of each piece.

Name the pieces of the internal structure of the female reproductive system, and explain the functions of each piece.

Name the pieces of the integumentary system, and name the three main functions of the integumentary system.

Explain the functions associated with protection, secretion, and communication in the integumentary system.

In addition to protection, secretion, and communication, what else can the integumentary system do?

The external portion of the female reproductive system includes the labia majora, labia minora, Bartholin's glands and clitoris.

The **labia majora** and the **labia minora** enclose and protect the vagina. The **Bartholin's glands** secrete a lubricating fluid. The **clitoris** contains erectile tissue and nerve endings for sensual pleasure.

The functions of the female reproductive system are to produce **ova** (oocytes, or egg cells), transfer the ova to the **fallopian tubes** for fertilization, receive the sperm from the male, and to provide a protective, nourishing environment for the developing **embryo**.

The **integumentary system**, which consists of the skin including the sebaceous glands sweat glands, hair, and nails, serves a variety of functions associated with protection, secretion, and communication.

The internal portion of the female reproductive system includes the ovaries, fallopian tubes, uterus, and vagina.

The **ovaries**, which are the female gonads, produce the ova and secrete **estrogen** and **progesterone**. The **fallopian tubes** carry the mature egg toward the uterus. Fertilization typically occurs in the fallopian tubes. If fertilized, the egg travels to the **uterus**, where it implants in the uterine wall. The uterus protects and nourishes the developing embryo until birth. The **vagina** is a muscular tube that extends from the **cervix** of the uterus to the outside of the body. The vagina receives the semen and sperm during sexual intercourse and provides a birth canal when needed.

In addition to protection, secretion, and communication, the skin manufactures **vitamin D** and can absorb certain chemicals such as specific medications.

In the functions associated with protection, the integumentary system protects the body from **pathogens** including bacteria, viruses, and various chemicals from entering the body.

In the functions associated with secretion, **sebaceous glands** secrete **sebum** (oil) that waterproofs the skin, and **sweat glands** are associated with the body's homeostatic relationship of **thermoregulation**. Sweat glands also serve as excretory organs and help rid the body of metabolic wastes.

In the functions associated with communication, **sensory receptors** distributed throughout the skin send information to the brain regarding pain, touch, pressure, and temperature.

Human Anatomy and Physiology
© Mometrix Media – flashcardsecrets.com/teas
ATI TEAS Science

Name the layers of skin in the human body, and explain some of the features of the epidermis and the deepest portion of the epidermis.

Human Anatomy and Physiology
© Mometrix Media – flashcardsecrets.com/teas
ATI TEAS Science

What happens as more and more skin cells are produced?

Human Anatomy and Physiology
© Mometrix Media – flashcardsecrets.com/teas
ATI TEAS Science

Name the location of the dermis and the contents of the dermis.

Human Anatomy and Physiology
© Mometrix Media – flashcardsecrets.com/teas
ATI TEAS Science

Name the layer that is not actually a layer of skin, and name the features of this layer.

Human Anatomy and Physiology
© Mometrix Media – flashcardsecrets.com/teas
ATI TEAS Science

What component of the human body is activated to assist in temperature homeostasis?

Human Anatomy and Physiology
© Mometrix Media – flashcardsecrets.com/teas
ATI TEAS Science

Name the parts and location of the negative feedback system that control the temperature of the body.

As more and more cells are produced, older cells are pushed toward the surface. Most epidermal cells are keratinized. **Keratin** is a waxy protein that helps to waterproof the skin. As the cells die, they are sloughed off.

The layers of the skin from the surface of the skin inward are the epidermis and dermis. The subcutaneous layer lying below the dermis is also part of the integumentary system.

The **epidermis** is the most superficial layer of the skin. The epidermis, which consists entirely of **epithelial cells**, does not contain any blood vessels.

The deepest portion of the epidermis is the **stratum basale**, which is a single layer of cells that continually undergo division.

The **subcutaneous layer** or **hypodermis** is actually not a layer of the skin.

The subcutaneous layer consists of connective tissue, which binds the skin to the underlying muscles. Fat deposits in the subcutaneous layer help to cushion and insulate the body.

The **dermis** lies directly beneath the epidermis. The dermis consists mostly of connective tissue. The dermis contains blood vessels, sensory receptors, hair follicles, sebaceous glands, and sweat glands. The dermis also contains **elastin** and **collagen fibers**.

The temperature of the body is controlled by a negative feedback system consisting of a receptor, control center, and effector.

The **receptors** are sensory cells located in the dermis of the skin.

The **control center** is the **hypothalamus**, which is located in the brain.

The **effectors** include the *sweat glands, blood vessels, and muscles*. The evaporation of sweat across the surface of the skin cools the body to maintain its tolerance range.

The skin is involved in **temperature homeostasis** or thermoregulation through the activation of the sweat glands.

By **thermoregulation**, the body maintains a stable body temperature as one component of a stable internal environment.

What is vasodilation and the role of muscles in thermoregulation?

Name two of the exocrine glands found in the skin, and name a responsibility of these exocrine glands.

What is the relationship between sebaceous glands and sebum?

Name the two types of glands that can be sweat glands, and explain the role, the location, and the features of eccrine glands.

Explain the role and the location of the apocrine glands.

Name the responsibility of the endocrine system, and name the parts of the human body that establish a working relationship between the endocrine system and the nervous system.

Sebaceous glands and sweat glands are exocrine glands found in the skin.

Exocrine glands secrete substances into **ducts**. In this case, the secretions are through the ducts to the surface of the skin.

Vasodilation of the blood vessels near the surface of the skin also releases heat into the environment to lower body temperature.

The muscles that are included with the effectors are partly responsible for shivering which is also associated with the muscular system.

Sweat glands are either eccrine glands or apocrine glands.

Eccrine glands are not connected to hair follicles. They are activated by elevated body temperature. Eccrine glands are located throughout the body and can be found on the forehead, neck, and back. Eccrine glands secrete a salty solution of electrolytes and water containing sodium chloride, potassium, bicarbonate, glucose, and antimicrobial peptides.

Eccrine glands are activated as part of the body's thermoregulation.

Sebaceous glands are **holocrine glands**, which secrete sebum.

Sebum is an oily mixture of lipids and proteins. Sebaceous glands are connected to hair follicles and secrete sebum through the hair pore. Sebum inhibits water loss from the skin and protects against bacterial and fungal infections.

The **endocrine system** is responsible for secreting the **hormones** and other molecules that help regulate the entire body in both the short and the long term.

There is a close working relationship between the endocrine system and the nervous system. The **hypothalamus** and the **pituitary gland** coordinate to serve as a **neuroendocrine control center**.

Apocrine glands secrete an oily solution containing fatty acids, triglycerides, and proteins. Apocrine glands are located in the armpits, groin, palms, and soles of the feet. Apocrine glands secrete this oily sweat when a person experiences stress or anxiety. Bacteria feed on apocrine sweat and expel aromatic fatty acids, producing body odor.

What are some of the signals that trigger hormone secretion?

What is the "key in the lock" model for hormonal action?

What is the role of steroid and protein hormones?

Give an example of a hormone that works quickly, and explain the results of slower acting hormones.

Name the eight major endocrine glands and their functions.

Name what is located amongst the groupings of exocrine cells, and name the contents of the islets of Langerhans.

Only cells with particular **receptors** can benefit from hormonal influence. This is the "key in the lock" model for hormonal action.

Hormone secretion is triggered by a variety of signals, including hormonal signs, chemical reactions, and environmental cues.

Hormones such as **insulin** work quickly when the body signals an urgent need. Slower acting hormones afford longer, gradual, and sometimes permanent changes in the body.

Steroid hormones trigger gene activation and protein synthesis in some target cells. **Protein hormones** change the activity of existing enzymes in target cells.

Located amongst the groupings of **exocrine cells** (acini) are groups of **endocrine cells** (called islets of Langerhans).

The **islets of Langerhans** are primarily made up of insulin-producing **beta cells** (fifty to eighty percent of the total) and glucagon-releasing **alpha cells**.

The eight major endocrine glands and their functions are:
- **Adrenal cortex** – Monitors blood sugar level; helps in lipid and protein metabolism.
- **Adrenal medulla** – Controls cardiac function; raises blood sugar and controls the size of blood vessels.
- **Thyroid gland** – Helps regulate metabolism and functions in growth and development.
- **Parathyroid** – Regulates calcium levels in the blood.
- **Pancreas islets** – Raises and lowers blood sugar; active in carbohydrate metabolism.
- **Thymus gland** – Plays a role in immune responses.
- **Pineal gland** – Has an influence on daily biorhythms and sexual activity.
- **Pituitary gland** – Plays an important role in growth and development.

Human Anatomy and Physiology
ATI TEAS Science

Name the two major hormones produced by the pancreas, and explain how the human body uses these major hormones.

Human Anatomy and Physiology
ATI TEAS Science

Why are the levels of insulin and glucagon balanced?

Human Anatomy and Physiology
ATI TEAS Science

Name the location of the thyroid gland and the parathyroid gland.

Human Anatomy and Physiology
ATI TEAS Science

Name the basic function of the thyroid gland. Then, name the hormones secreted by the thyroid gland and what role those hormones play.

Human Anatomy and Physiology
ATI TEAS Science

What is the role of the hypothalamus and the parathyroid glands?

Human Anatomy and Physiology
ATI TEAS Science

Name the capability of the urinary system and the main parts of this system.

The levels of insulin and glucagon are balanced to maintain the optimum level of blood sugar (glucose) throughout the day.

The major hormones produced by the pancreas are insulin and glucagon.

The body uses **insulin** to control carbohydrate metabolism by lowering the amount of sugar (**glucose**) in the blood. Insulin also affects fat **metabolism** and can change the liver's ability to release stored fat.

The body also uses **glucagon** to control carbohydrate metabolism. Glucagon has the opposite effect of insulin in that the body uses it to increase blood sugar (glucose) levels.

The basic function of the **thyroid gland** is to regulate metabolism.

The thyroid gland secretes the hormones thyroxine, triiodothyronine, and calcitonin.

Thyroxine and **triiodothyronine** increase metabolism, and **calcitonin** decreases blood calcium by storing calcium in bone tissue.

The **thyroid** and **parathyroid glands** are located in the neck just below the larynx. The parathyroid glands are four small glands that are embedded on the posterior side of the thyroid gland.

The **urinary system** is capable of eliminating excess substances while preserving the substances needed by the body to function.

The urinary system consists of the kidneys, urinary ducts, and bladder.

The **hypothalamus** directs the pituitary gland to secrete **thyroid-stimulating hormone** (TSH), which stimulates the thyroid gland to release these hormones as needed via a negative-feedback mechanism.

The **parathyroid glands** secrete **parathyroid hormone**, which can increase blood calcium by moving calcium from the bone to the blood.

Name the shape, location, and the three layers of the kidneys.

Name the "tiny, individual" filters of the kidneys, and explain what each of those filters contains.

What is the pathway that blood takes from when the kidneys receive blood to when organic molecules are reabsorbed into the bloodstream?

What happens to materials in the kidneys that are removed from the bloodstream?

Name the main function of the immune system and the main parts of the immune system.

Explain some of the key roles of the lymphatic system within the immune system, and name the location of the lymph nodes.

The **kidneys** are bean-shaped structures that are located at the back of the abdominal cavity just under the diaphragm.

Each kidney consists of three layers: the renal cortex (outer layer), renal medulla (inner layer), and renal pelvis (innermost portion).

The **renal cortex** is composed of approximately one million **nephrons**, which are the tiny, individual filters of the kidneys. Each nephron contains a cluster of capillaries called a **glomerulus** surrounded by the cup-shaped **Bowman's capsule**, which leads to a tubule.

The kidneys receive blood from the **renal arteries**, which branch off the aorta. In general, the kidneys filter the blood, reabsorb needed materials, and secrete wastes and excess water in the urine.

More specifically, blood flows from the renal arteries into **arterioles** into the glomerulus, where it is filtered. The **glomerular filtrate** enters the **proximal convoluted tub**ule where water, glucose, ions, and other organic molecules are reabsorbed back into the bloodstream.

Additional substances such as urea and drugs are removed from the blood in the **distal convoluted tubule**. Also, the pH of the blood can be adjusted in the distal convoluted tubule by the secretion of **hydrogen ions**.

Finally, the unabsorbed materials flow out from the collecting tubules located in the **renal medulla** to the **renal pelvis** as urine.

Urine is drained from the kidneys through the **ureters** to the **urinary bladder**, where it is stored until expulsion from the body through the **urethra**.

The immune system protects the body against invading **pathogens** including bacteria, viruses, fungi, and protists.

The immune system includes the **lymphatic system** (lymph, lymph capillaries, lymph vessel, and lymph nodes) as well as the **red bone marrow** and numerous **leukocytes**, or white blood cells.

Tissue fluid enters the **lymph capillaries**, which combine to form **lymph vessels**.

Skeletal muscle contractions move the lymph one way through the lymphatic system to lymphatic ducts, which dump back into the venous blood supply into the **lymph nodes**, which are situated along the lymph vessels, and filter the lymph of pathogens and other matter.

The lymph nodes are concentrated in the neck, armpits, and groin areas.

Name the parts of the immune system that are outside the lymphatic vessel system, and describe the role of each part.

Name the parts of the human body's general immune defenses, and name the responsibility of each part.

Name the responses that mobilize white blood cells and chemical reactions to stop infection and the proteins that act as a complement to repel bacteria and pathogens.

Name the three types of white blood cells that form the foundation of the human body's immune system, and name three other cells that contribute to the body's defense.

Explain the difference between immune responses that are anti-body mediated and cell-mediated, and note when these responses recede.

What is a secondary immune response?

The body's general immune defenses include:
- **Skin** – An intact epidermis and dermis form a formidable barrier against bacteria.
- **Ciliated Mucous Membranes** – Cilia sweep pathogens out of the respiratory tract.
- **Glandular Secretions** – Secretions from exocrine glands destroy bacteria.
- **Gastric Secretions** – Gastric acid destroys pathogens.
- **Normal Bacterial Populations** – Compete with pathogens in the gut and vagina.

Outside the lymphatic vessel system lies the **lymphatic tissue** including the tonsils, adenoids, thymus, spleen, and Peyer's patches.

The **tonsils**, located in the pharynx, protect against pathogens entering the body through the mouth and throat. The **thymus** serves as a maturation chamber for the immature T cells that are formed in the bone marrow. The **spleen** cleans the blood of dead cells and pathogens. **Peyer's patches**, which are located in the small intestine, protect the digestive system from pathogens.

Three types of white blood cells form the foundation of the body's immune system. They are:
- **Macrophages** – Phagocytes that alert T cells to the presence of foreign substances.
- **T Lymphocytes** – These directly attack cells infected by viruses and bacteria.
- **B Lymphocytes** – These cells target specific bacteria for destruction.

Memory cells, **suppressor T cells**, and **helper T cells** also contribute to the body's defense.

Phagocytes and inflammation responses mobilize white blood cells and chemical reactions to stop infection. These responses include localized redness, tissue repair, and fluid-seeping healing agents.

Additionally, **plasma proteins** act as the complement system to repel bacteria and pathogens.

Once an invader has attacked the body, if it returns it is immediately recognized and a secondary immune response occurs. This secondary response is rapid and powerful, much more so than the original response. These memory lymphocytes circulate throughout the body for years, alert to a possible new attack.

Immune responses can be **antibody-mediated** when the response is to an antigen, or **cell-mediated** when the response is to already infected cells.

These responses are controlled and measured counter-attacks that recede when the foreign agents are destroyed.

Name where leukocytes are produced, and name how they can be classified.

Explain the features and roles of specific monocytes and granulocytes.

Name the purpose of each kind of T cell, and name the purpose of B cells.

Give a definition of antigens, name their typical location, and list some substances that can also be antigens.

Name the body's reaction to unfamiliar antigens, and name what specific antibodies are produced for.

Explain the roles of macrophages, helper T cells, and killer T cells in a typical immune response.

Macrophages found traveling in the lymph or fixed in lymphatic tissue are the largest, long-living phagocytes that engulf and destroy pathogens. **Dendritic cells** present antigens (foreign particles) to T cells.

Neutrophils are short-living phagocytes that respond quickly to invaders. **Basophils** alert the body of invasion. **Eosinophils** are large, long-living phagocytes that defend against multicellular invaders.

Antigens are substances that stimulate the **immune system**. Antigens are typically proteins on the surfaces of bacteria, viruses, and fungi.

Substances such as drugs, toxins, and foreign particles can also be antigens.

In a typical immune response, when a pathogen or foreign substance enters the body, it is engulfed by a **macrophage**, which presents fragments of the antigen on its surface.

A **helper T cell** joins the macrophage, and the killer (cytotoxic) T cells and B cells are activated. **Killer T cells** search out and destroy cells presenting the same antigens.

Leukocytes, or white blood cells, are produced in the red bone marrow.

Leukocytes can be classified as **monocytes** (macrophages and dendritic cells), **granulocytes** (neutrophils, basophils, and eosinophils), **T lymphocytes, B lymphocytes**, or **natural killer cells**.

T lymphocytes or T cells include helper T cells, killer T cells, suppressor T cells, and memory T cells.

Helper T cells help the body fight infections by producing antibodies and other chemicals.

Killer T cells destroy cells that are infected with a virus or pathogen and tumor cells.

Suppressor T cells stop or "suppress" the other T cells when the battle is over.

Memory T cells remain in the blood on alert in case the invader attacks again.

B lymphocytes, or B cells, produce antibodies.

The human body recognizes the antigens of its own cells, but it will attack cells or substances with unfamiliar antigens.

Specific **antibodies** are produced for each antigen that enters the body.

What is the role of B cells and antibodies in a typical immune response?

What is an adaptive immunity?

Explain the difference between an acquired active immunity that is natural and one that is artificial.

Define an artificially acquired passive immunity, and explain the purpose of such an immunity.

Name the main division of the skeletal structure.

Name the parts of the axial skeleton, and note the primary purpose of the axial skeleton.

At birth, an **innate immune system** protects an individual from pathogens. When an individual encounters infection or has an immunization, the individual develops an **adaptive immunity** that reacts to pathogens. So, this adaptive immunity is acquired.

B cells differentiate into plasma cells and memory cells.

Plasma cells produce antibodies specific to that pathogen or foreign substance.

Antibodies bind to antigens on the surface of pathogens and mark them for destruction by other phagocytes.

Memory cells remain in the blood stream to protect against future infections from the same pathogen.

An **artificially acquired passive immunity** is an *immunization* that is given in recent outbreaks or emergency situations.

This immunization provides quick and short-lived protection to disease by the use of antibodies that can come from another person or animal.

A **naturally acquired active immunity** is natural because the individual is exposed and builds immunity to a pathogen *without an immunization*.

An **artificially acquired active immunity** is artificial because the individual is exposed and builds immunity to a pathogen *by a vaccine*.

The **axial skeleton** consists of 80 bones and includes the vertebral column, rib cage, sternum, skull, and hyoid bone.

The **vertebral column** consists of 33 vertebrae classified as cervical vertebrae, thoracic vertebrae, lumbar vertebrae, and sacral vertebrae. The **rib cage** includes 12 paired ribs, 10 pairs of true ribs and 2 pairs of floating ribs, and the **sternum**, which consists of the manubrium, corpus sterni, and xiphoid process.

The **skull** includes the cranium and facial bones. The **ossicles** are bones in the middle ear. The **hyoid bone** provides an attachment point for the tongue muscles.

The axial skeleton protects vital organs including the brain, heart, and lungs.

The **skeletal structure** in humans contains both **bones** and **cartilage**. Over 200 bones in the human body can be divided into two parts:
- **Axial skeleton** – Includes the skull, sternum, ribs, and vertebral column (the spine).
- **Appendicular skeleton** – Includes the bones of the arms, feet, hands, legs, hips, and shoulders.

Name the parts of the appendicular skeleton.

What are some of the basic functions of the skeletal system?

The axial skeleton transfers the weight from the upper body to what part of the body?

How does the skeletal system provide movement with joints and the muscular system?

Name the parts of the human skeletal system that protect the brain, the spinal cord, the heart and lungs, and the reproductive organs.

What are the roles of red marrow and yellow marrow in the human body?

The **skeletal system** serves many functions including providing structural support, providing movement, providing protection, producing blood cells, and storing substances such as fat and minerals.

The skeletal system provides the body with structure and support for the muscles and organs.

The skeletal system provides movement with **joints** and the muscular system.

Bones provide attachment points for muscles. Joints including **hinge joints**, ball-and-socket joints, **pivot joints, ellipsoid joints, gliding joints,** and **saddle joints**.

Each muscle is attached to two bones: the origin and the insertion. The **origin** remains immobile, and the **insertion** is the bone that moves as the muscle contracts and relaxes.

The **red marrow** manufactures red and white blood cells. All bone marrow is red at birth, but adults have approximately one-half red bone marrow and one-half yellow bone marrow. **Yellow bone marrow** stores fat.

The **appendicular skeleton** consists of 126 bones including the pectoral girdle, pelvic girdle, and appendages.

The **pectoral girdle** consists of the scapulae (shoulders) and clavicles (collarbones). The **pelvic girdle** consists of two pelvic (hip) bones, which attach to the sacrum.

The **upper appendages** (arms) include the humerus, radius, ulna, carpals, metacarpals, and phalanges. The **lower appendages** (legs) include the femur, patella, fibula, tibia, tarsals, metatarsals, and phalanges.

The axial skeleton transfers the weight from the upper body to the lower appendages.

The skeletal system serves to protect the body.

The **cranium** protects the brain. The **vertebrae** protect the spinal cord. The **rib cage** protects the heart and lungs. The **pelvis** protects the reproductive organs.

Human Anatomy and Physiology
© Mometrix Media – flashcardsecrets.com/teas
ATI TEAS Science

What are two minerals that can be stored in a reservoir by the skeletal system?

Human Anatomy and Physiology
© Mometrix Media – flashcardsecrets.com/teas
ATI TEAS Science

Explain the roles of movement, mineral storage, support, protection, and blood cell formation within the skeletal system.

Human Anatomy and Physiology
© Mometrix Media – flashcardsecrets.com/teas
ATI TEAS Science

Name the three ways that bones can be classified, and explain what bones are made of and the frequency and importance of bone regeneration.

Human Anatomy and Physiology
© Mometrix Media – flashcardsecrets.com/teas
ATI TEAS Science

Explain the features and structure of the human backbone, and review some of the consequences of trauma or shock to the backbone.

Human Anatomy and Physiology
© Mometrix Media – flashcardsecrets.com/teas
ATI TEAS Science

Explain the roles of synovial joints, cartilaginous joints, and fibrous joints, and name the two types of connective bone tissue.

Human Anatomy and Physiology
© Mometrix Media – flashcardsecrets.com/teas
ATI TEAS Science

Explain the features and structure of compact bone, and explain the role of the Haversian system.

The skeletal system has an important role in the following body functions:
- **Movement** – The action of skeletal muscles on bones moves the body.
- **Mineral Storage** – Bones serve as storage facilities for essential mineral ions.
- **Support** – Bones act as a framework and support system for the organs.
- **Protection** – Bones surround and protect key organs in the body.
- **Blood Cell Formation** – Red blood cells are produced in the marrow of certain bones.

The skeletal system provides a reservoir to store the minerals **calcium** and **phosphorus**.

The flexible and curved **backbone** is supported by muscles and ligaments. **Intervertebral discs** are stacked one above another and provide cushioning for the backbone.

Trauma or shock may cause these discs to **herniate** and cause pain. The sensitive **spinal cord** is enclosed in a cavity which is well protected by the bones of the vertebrae.

Bones are classified as long, short, flat, or irregular.

Bones are a connective tissue with a base of pulp containing **collagen** and living cells.

Bone tissue is constantly regenerating itself as the mineral composition changes. This allows for special needs during growth periods and maintains calcium levels for the body.

Bone regeneration can deteriorate in old age, particularly among women, leading to **osteoporosis**.

Compact, or **cortical**, bone, which consists of tightly packed cells, is strong, dense, and rigid. Running vertically throughout compact bone are the **Haversian canals**, which are surrounded by concentric circles of bone tissue called **lamellae**.

The spaces between the lamellae are called the **lacunae**. These lamellae and canals along with their associated arteries, veins, lymph vessels, and nerve endings are referred to collectively as the **Haversian system**.

The Haversian system provides a reservoir for calcium and phosphorus for the blood.

Joints are areas of contact adjacent to bones.

- **Synovial joints** are the most common, and are freely moveable. These may be found at the shoulders and knees.
- **Cartilaginous joints** fill the spaces between some bones and restrict movement. Examples of cartilaginous joints are those between vertebrae.
- **Fibrous joints** have fibrous tissue connecting bones and no cavity is present.

Two types of connective bone tissue include compact bone and spongy bone.

Human Anatomy and Physiology
© Mometrix Media – flashcardsecrets.com/teas
ATI TEAS Science

What gives bones their characteristic smooth, white appearance?

Human Anatomy and Physiology
© Mometrix Media – flashcardsecrets.com/teas
ATI TEAS Science

Explain the contents of spongy bone, and explain how spongy bone is different from compact bone.

Human Anatomy and Physiology
© Mometrix Media – flashcardsecrets.com/teas
ATI TEAS Science

What are the contents of the diaphysis?

Life and Physical Sciences
© Mometrix Media – flashcardsecrets.com/teas
ATI TEAS Science

Describe macromolecules, and name their role. Then, name the four basic organic macromolecules produced by anabolic reactions, and name the four basic building blocks involved in catabolic reactions.

Life and Physical Sciences
© Mometrix Media – flashcardsecrets.com/teas
ATI TEAS Science

What are the differences among anabolic, catabolic, and endothermic reactions?

Life and Physical Sciences
© Mometrix Media – flashcardsecrets.com/teas
ATI TEAS Science

Name the responsibility of carbohydrates, name what provides cells with most of their energy, and name the metabolic energy cycles that involve carbohydrates.

Spongy, or **cancellous**, bone consists of **trabeculae**, which are a network of girders with open spaces filled with red bone marrow.

Compared to compact bone, spongy bone is lightweight and porous, which helps reduce the bone's overall weight.

Bones have a thin outside layer of compact bone, which gives them their characteristic smooth, white appearance.

Macromolecules are large and complex, and play an important role in cell structure and function.

The four basic organic macromolecules produced by anabolic reactions are **carbohydrates** (polysaccharides), **nucleic acids**, **proteins**, and **lipids**.

The four basic building blocks involved in catabolic reactions are **monosaccharides** (glucose), **amino acids**, **fatty acids** (glycerol), and **nucleotides**.

In long bones, the **diaphysis** consists of compact bone surrounding the marrow cavity and spongy bone containing red marrow in the **epiphyses**.

Carbohydrates are the primary source of energy and are responsible for providing energy as they can be easily converted to **glucose**. Glucose can be further broken down by respiration or fermentation by **glycolysis**.

It is the oxidation of carbohydrates that provides the cells with most of their energy. They are involved in the metabolic energy cycles of photosynthesis and respiration.

An **anabolic reaction** is one that builds larger and more complex molecules (macromolecules) from smaller ones. **Catabolic reactions** are the opposite. Larger molecules are broken down into smaller, simpler molecules. Catabolic reactions *release energy*, while anabolic ones *require energy*.

Endothermic reactions are chemical reactions that *absorb* heat and **exothermic reactions** are chemical reactions that *release* heat.

Life and Physical Sciences
© Mometrix Media – flashcardsecrets.com/teas
ATI TEAS Science

Explain the chemical structure of carbohydrates, and name the two things that follow from carbohydrates being broken down.

Life and Physical Sciences
© Mometrix Media – flashcardsecrets.com/teas
ATI TEAS Science

Name the two categories of simple sugars, and explain their differences.

Life and Physical Sciences
© Mometrix Media – flashcardsecrets.com/teas
ATI TEAS Science

Explain the difference between monomers and polymers, and name some of the members that are polymers.

Life and Physical Sciences
© Mometrix Media – flashcardsecrets.com/teas
ATI TEAS Science

Explain the features of lipids, name the major roles of lipids, and give some examples of lipids.

Life and Physical Sciences
© Mometrix Media – flashcardsecrets.com/teas
ATI TEAS Science

Explain the features and structure of fats, and give an example that contains the sodium salts of free fatty acids.

Life and Physical Sciences
© Mometrix Media – flashcardsecrets.com/teas
ATI TEAS Science

Name the difference in the structure of phospholipids and glycerides, and give some examples of glycerides.

The simple sugars can be grouped into monosaccharides (glucose, fructose, and galactose) and disaccharides. These are both types of carbohydrates.

Monosaccharides have one monomer of sugar and disaccharides have two.

Monosaccharides (CH_2O) have one carbon for every water molecule.

Structurally, carbohydrates usually take the form of some variation of CH_2O as they are made of carbon, hydrogen, and oxygen.

Carbohydrates (**polysaccharides**) are broken down into sugars or glucose.

Lipids are molecules that are soluble in nonpolar solvents, but are hydrophobic, meaning they do not bond well with water or mix well with water solutions. Lipids have numerous **C–H bonds**. In this way, they are similar to **hydrocarbons** (substances consisting only of carbon and hydrogen).

The major roles of lipids include energy storage and structural functions. Examples of lipids include fats, phospholipids, steroids, and waxes.

A **monomer** is a small molecule. It is a single compound that forms chemical bonds with other monomers to make a polymer. A **polymer** is a compound of large molecules formed by repeating monomers.

Carbohydrates, proteins, and nucleic acids are groups of macromolecules that are polymers.

Phospholipids are lipids that have a phosphate group rather than a fatty acid.

Glycerides are another type of lipid. Glycerides are formed from fatty acids and glycerol (a type of alcohol). Examples of glycerides are fat and oil.

Fats (which are triglycerides) are made of long chains of fatty acids (three fatty acids bound to a glycerol). **Fatty acids** are chains with reduced carbon at one end and a carboxylic acid group at the other. An example is soap, which contains the sodium salts of free fatty acids.

Life and Physical Sciences

Explain the structure of proteins.

Life and Physical Sciences

Explain the difference between a condensation reaction and a hydrolysis reaction.

Life and Physical Sciences

What is involved to form amino acids?

Life and Physical Sciences

Define *enzymes*, and explain their influence on chemical reactions.

Life and Physical Sciences

How does the "key in the lock" analogy apply to enzymes?

Life and Physical Sciences

What is the unusual quality of enzymes with respect to chemical reactions?

A **condensation reaction** results in a loss of water when two molecules are joined together. A **hydrolysis reaction** is the opposite of a condensation reaction.

During hydrolysis, water is added. –H is added to one of the smaller molecules and OH is added to another molecule being formed.

Proteins are macromolecules formed from amino acids. They are **polypeptides**, which consist of many (10 to 100) peptides linked together. The peptide connections are the result of condensation reactions.

Enzymes are proteins with strong **catalytic** power.

They greatly accelerate the speed at which specific reactions approach equilibrium. Although enzymes do not start chemical reactions that would not eventually occur by themselves, they do make these reactions happen faster and more often. This acceleration can be substantial, sometimes making reactions happen a million times faster.

A **peptide** is a compound of two or more amino acids. **Amino acids** are formed by the partial hydrolysis of protein, which forms an **amide bond**.

This partial hydrolysis involves an amine group and a carboxylic acid. In the carbon chain of amino acids, there is a **carboxylic acid group** (–COOH), an **amine group** (–NH$_2$), a **central carbon atom** between them with an attached hydrogen, and an attached **"R" group** (side chain), which is different for different amino acids.

It is the "R" group that determines the properties of the protein.

An unusual quality of enzymes is that they are not permanently consumed in the reactions they speed up. They can be used again and again, providing a constant source of energy accelerators for cells. This allows for a tremendous increase in the number and rate of reactions in cells.

Each type of enzyme deals with **reactants**, also called **substrates**. Each enzyme is highly selective, only interacting with substrates that are a match for it at an active site on the enzyme. This is the "key in the lock" analogy: a certain enzyme only fits with certain substrates. Even with a matching substrate, an enzyme must sometimes reshape itself to fit well with the substrate, forming a strong bond that aids in catalyzing a reaction before it returns to its original shape.

Define *nucleic acids*, and explain the process that breaks down nucleic acids to make oligonucleotides.

Explain the steps of the process that takes oligonucleotides and leads to the formation of the five types of nitrogenous bases.

Name the bonds that hold the monomeric units of nucleotides, and name what cells need to synthesize proteins from amino acids and replicate DNA.

What is nitrogen fixation?

Explain the role of nucleic acids, name the item that catalyzes the transfer of DNA genetic information, and name what is considered to be an RNA nucleotide.

Explain the role and the structure of nucleotides.

Oligonucleotides are broken down into smaller sugar nitrogenous units called **nucleosides**. These can be digested by cells since the sugar is divided from the nitrogenous base.

This, in turn, leads to the formation of the five types of nitrogenous bases, sugars, and the preliminary substances involved in the synthesis of new RNA and DNA. DNA and RNA have a helix shape.

Nucleic acids are macromolecules that are composed of **nucleotides**.

Hydrolysis is a reaction in which water is broken down into **hydrogen cations** (H or H$^+$) and **hydroxide anions** (OH or OH$^-$). This is part of the process by which nucleic acids are broken down by enzymes to produce shorter strings of RNA and DNA (oligonucleotides).

Nitrogen fixation is used to synthesize nucleotides for DNA and amino acids for proteins. Nitrogen fixation uses the enzyme nitrogenase in the reduction of dinitrogen gas (N_2) to ammonia (NH_3).

Macromolecular nucleic acid polymers, such as RNA and DNA, are formed from nucleotides, which are monomeric units joined by **phosphodiester bonds**.

Cells require energy in the form of ATP to synthesize proteins from amino acids and replicate DNA.

Nucleotides are used to form the nucleic acids. Nucleotides are made of a five carbon sugar, such as ribose or deoxyribose, a nitrogenous base, and one or more phosphates. Nucleotides consisting of more than one phosphate can also store energy in their bonds.

Nucleic acids store information and energy and are also important catalysts.

It is the **RNA** that catalyzes the transfer of **DNA genetic information** into protein coded information.

ATP is an RNA nucleotide.

Explain the location and name the role of DNA.

Describe the structure of DNA, and explain how this model of the structure was discovered and developed.

What are the contents of DNA?

Name the four nitrogenous bases of DNA, explain the role of the nitrogenous bases of DNA, and explain the role that these bases have played in human diversity.

What are the differences between pyrimidine bases and purine bases?

Describe nucleosides, and give some examples.

The model or structure of DNA is described as a **double helix**. A helix is a curve, and a double helix is two congruent curves connected by horizontal members. The model can be likened to a spiral staircase. It is right-handed.

The British scientist Rosalind Elsie Franklin is credited with taking the x-ray diffraction image in 1952 that was used by Francis Crick and James Watson to formulate the double-helix model of DNA and speculate about its important role in carrying and transferring genetic information.

Chromosomes consist of **genes**, which are single units of genetic information. Genes are made up of deoxyribonucleic acid (DNA).

DNA is a nucleic acid located in the cell nucleus. There is also DNA in the **mitochondria**. DNA replicates to pass on genetic information. The DNA in almost all cells is the same. It is also involved in the biosynthesis of proteins.

The bases are attached to each other with hydrogen bonds, which are easily dismantled so replication can occur. Each base is attached to a phosphate and to a sugar. There are four types of nitrogenous bases: **adenine** (A), **guanine** (G), **cytosine** (C), and **thymine** (T).

There are about 3 billion bases in human DNA. The bases are mostly the same in everybody, but their order is different. It is the order of these bases that creates diversity in people. Adenine (A) pairs with thymine (T), and cytosine (C) pairs with guanine (G).

DNA has a double helix shape, resembles a twisted ladder, and is compact. It consists of **nucleotides**. Nucleotides consist of a **five-carbon sugar** (pentose), a **phosphate group**, and a **nitrogenous base**. Two bases pair up to form the rungs of the ladder. The "side rails" or backbone consists of the covalently bonded sugar and phosphate.

When combined with a sugar, any of the five bases become **nucleosides**. Nucleosides formed from purine bases end in "osine" and those formed from pyrimidine bases end in "idine." **Adenosine** and **thymidine** are examples of nucleosides.

The five bases in DNA and RNA can be categorized as either pyrimidine or purine according to their structure. The **pyrimidine bases** include cytosine, thymine, and uracil. They are six-sided and have a single ring shape. The **purine bases** are adenine and guanine, which consist of two attached rings. One ring has five sides and the other has six.

List the order of components of genes starting with the most basic and ending with the most complex.

Explain how codons can be visualized, and name the number of codons in relation to the number of amino acids.

Name what can be used to synthesize the necessary amino acids, and give examples of what can serve as codons for lysine.

Read the following string, and research what the following codons are in this string: AAAUCUUCGU.

If the string of codons below were read in groups of three starting from the second letter in the series, what would be the difference from starting at the first letter?
AAAUCUUCGU.

What are the start and stop codons?

Codons are groups of three nucleotides on the messenger RNA, and can be visualized as three rungs of a ladder. A codon has the code for a single amino acid.

There are 64 codons but 20 amino acids.

Bases are the most basic components, followed by nucleosides, nucleotides, and then DNA or RNA.

These groups of three occur in strings, and might be thought of as frames.

For example, AAAUCUUCGU, if read in groups of three from the beginning, would be AAA, UCU, UCG, which are codons for lysine, serine, and serine, respectively.

More than one combination, or triplet, can be used to synthesize the necessary amino acids. For example, AAA (adenine-adenine-adenine) or AAG (adenine-adenine-guanine) can serve as codons for lysine.

There are **start** and **stop codons** that indicate the beginning and ending of a sequence (or frame). **AUG** (methionine) is the start codon. **UAA**, **UGA**, and **UAG**, also known as ocher, opal, and amber, respectively, are stop codons.

If the same sequence was read in groups of three starting from the second position, the groups would be AAU (asparagine), CUU (proline), and so on. The resulting amino acids would be completely different.

Name what happens to DNA when replication begins, and name what controls the steps of DNA replication.

Explain the steps of DNA replication.

Name the role of RNA and the types of RNA, and name what can use RNA to carry its genetic material to DNA.

What are the roles of ribosomal RNA and messenger RNA?

What are the roles of transcription, translation, and transfer RNA?

What are the differences between RNA and DNA in terms of *structure*?

The enzyme **helicase** instigates the deforming of hydrogen bonds between the bases to split the two strands. The splitting starts at the A-T bases (adenine and thymine) as there are only two hydrogen bonds.

The cytosine-guanine base pair has three bonds. The term **"origin of replication"** is used to refer to where the splitting starts. The portion of the DNA that is unwound to be replicated is called the **replication fork**. Each strand of DNA is transcribed by an mRNA. It copies the DNA onto itself, base by base, in a complementary manner. The exception is that uracil replaces thymine.

Pairs of chromosomes are composed of DNA, which is tightly wound to conserve space. When replication starts, it unwinds.

The steps in **DNA replication** are controlled by enzymes.

Ribosomal RNA is not believed to have changed much over time. For this reason, it can be used to study relationships in organisms.

Messenger RNA carries a copy of a strand of DNA and transports it from the nucleus to the cytoplasm.

RNA acts as a *helper* to DNA and carries out a number of other functions. Types of RNA include ribosomal RNA (rRNA), transfer RNA (tRNA), and messenger RNA (mRNA).

Viruses can use RNA to carry their genetic material to DNA.

RNA has a different sugar than DNA. It has **ribose** rather than **deoxyribose** sugar.

The RNA nitrogenous bases are adenine (A), guanine (G), cytosine (C), and uracil (U). **Uracil** is found only in RNA and **thymine** in found only in DNA. RNA consists of a single strand and DNA has two strands.

If straightened out, DNA has two side rails. RNA only has one "backbone," or strand of sugar and phosphate group components.

Transcription is the process in which RNA polymerase copies DNA into RNA. DNA unwinds itself and serves as a template while RNA is being assembled. The DNA molecules are copied to RNA.

Translation is the process whereby ribosomes use transcribed RNA to put together the needed protein.

Transfer RNA is a molecule that helps in the translation process, and is found in the cytoplasm. Ribosomal RNA is in the ribosomes.

What are the differences between RNA and DNA in terms of *function*?

Explain the law of segregation and the law of independent assortment.

Explain what a Punnett square can be used to illustrate and to predict.

Define *gene*, and give a brief explanation of the role that genes have in the human body.

What is the difference between genotypes and phenotypes?

Define *alleles*, and explain how eye color can be an example of the variations in genes.

The **law of segregation** states that there are two **alleles** and that half of the total number of alleles are contributed by each parent organism.

The **law of independent assortment** states that traits are passed on randomly and are not influenced by other traits. The exception to this is linked traits.

RNA uses the fully hydroxylated sugar **pentose**, which includes an extra oxygen compared to deoxyribose, which is the sugar used by DNA.

RNA supports the functions carried out by DNA. It aids in gene expression, replication, and transportation.

A **gene** is a portion of DNA that identifies how traits are expressed and passed on in an organism. A gene is part of the **genetic code**. Collectively, all genes form the **genotype** of an individual.

A **Punnett square** can illustrate how alleles combine from the contributing genes to form various **phenotypes**.

One set of a parent's genes are put in columns, while the genes from the other parent are placed in rows. The allele combinations are shown in each cell. When two different alleles are present in a pair, the **dominant** one is expressed.

A Punnett square can be used to predict the outcome of crosses.

An **allele** is a variation of a gene. Also known as a trait, it determines the manifestation of a gene. This manifestation results in a specific physical appearance of some facet of an organism, such as eye color or height.

For example, the genetic information for eye color is a gene. The gene variations responsible for blue, green, brown, or black eyes are called alleles. **Locus** (pl. loci) refers to the location of a gene or alleles.

The genotype includes genes that may not be expressed, such as **recessive genes**.

The **phenotype** is the physical, visual manifestation of genes. It is determined by the basic genetic information and how genes have been affected by their environment.

Explain how gene traits are represented, and explain why gene traits occur in pairs.

What is necessary in a gene pair for a trait to be dominant or recessive?

Define *monohybrid cross*, and explain the ratio of dominant gene manifestation to recessive gene manifestation.

What happens if one parent has a pair of dominant genes (DD) and the other has a pair of recessive (dd) genes?

Define *dihybrid crosses*, name the ratio of genotypes for a dihybrid cross when the traits are not linked, and name the ratio for incomplete dominance.

What will be the result in a Punnett square of a pea plant with green pods (G) and yellow pods (g) where pod color is homozygous?

A **dominant trait** only requires one gene of a gene pair for it to be expressed in a **phenotype**, whereas a **recessive** requires both genes in order to be manifested. For example, if the mother's genotype is Dd and the father's is dd, the possible combinations are Dd and dd.

The dominant trait will be manifested if the genotype is DD or Dd. The recessive trait will be manifested if the genotype is dd. Both DD and dd are **homozygous** pairs. Dd is **heterozygous**.

Gene traits are represented in pairs with an uppercase letter for the dominant trait (A) and a lowercase letter for the recessive trait (a).

Genes occur in pairs (AA, Aa, or aa). There is one gene on each chromosome half supplied by each parent organism. Since half the genetic material is from each parent, the offspring's traits are represented as a combination of these.

If one parent has a pair of dominant genes (DD) and the other has a pair of recessive (dd) genes, the recessive trait cannot be expressed in the next generation because the resulting crosses all have the Dd genotype.

A **monohybrid cross** refers to a cross involving only one trait. Typically, the ratio is 3:1 (DD, Dd, Dd, dd), which is the ratio of dominant gene manifestation to recessive gene manifestation. This ratio occurs when both parents have a pair of dominant and recessive genes.

For example, in pea plants, green pods (G) are dominant over yellow pods (g). In a genetic cross of two pea plants that are **homozygous** for pod color, the F_1 generation will be 100% heterozygous green pods.

	g	g
G	Gg	Gg
G	Gg	Gg

A **dihybrid cross** refers to one involving more than one trait, which means more combinations are possible.

The ratio of genotypes for a dihybrid cross is 9:3:3:1 when the traits are not linked.

The ratio for incomplete dominance is 1:2:1, which corresponds to dominant, mixed, and recessive phenotypes.

In a genetic cross of two pea plants that are homozygous for pod color and seed color, what will be the result in the F_1 generation?

If the F_1 pea plants that are 100% heterozygous green pods and yellow pods (GgYy) are crossed, what will the resulting F_2 generation be?

Define *co-dominance*, and give a couple of examples of co-dominance.

Define *incomplete dominance*.

Explain how snapdragons being red, white, or pink flowers make them a good example of incomplete dominance.

What is polygenic inheritance?

In pea plants, green pods (G) are dominant over yellow pods (g), and yellow seeds (Y) are dominant over green seeds (y).

In a genetic cross of two pea plants that are homozygous for pod color and seed color, the F_1 generation will be 100% heterozygous green pods and yellow seeds (GgYy).

If these F_1 plants are crossed, the resulting F_2 generation is shown below. There are nine genotypes for green-pod, yellow-seed plants: one GGYY, two GGYy, two GgYY, and four GgYy. There are three genotypes for green-pod, green-seed plants: one GGyy and two Ggyy. There are three genotypes for yellow-pod, yellow-seed plants: one ggYY and two ggYy. There is only one genotype for yellow-pod, green-seed plants: ggyy. This cross has a 9:3:3:1 ratio.

	GY	Gy	gY	gy
GY	GGYY	GGYy	GgYY	GgYy
Gy	GGYy	GGyy	GgYy	Ggyy
gY	GgYY	GgYy	ggYY	ggYy
gy	GgYy	Ggyy	ggYy	ggyy

Incomplete dominance is when both the **dominant** and **recessive** genes are expressed, resulting in a phenotype that is a mixture of the two.

Co-dominance refers to the expression of *both alleles* so that both traits are shown.

Cows, for example, can have hair colors of red, white, or red and white (not pink). In the latter color, both traits are fully expressed.

The ABO human blood typing system is also co-dominant.

Polygenic inheritance goes beyond the simplistic Mendelian concept that one gene influences one trait. It refers to traits that are influenced by *more than one gene*, and takes into account environmental influences on development.

The dominant red gene (RR) results in a red flower because of large amounts of red pigment.

White (rr) occurs because both genes call for no pigment. Pink (Rr) occurs because one gene is for red and one is for no pigment.

The colors blend to produce pink flowers. A cross of pink flowers (Rr) can result in red (RR), white (rr), or pink (Rr) flowers.

What is a multiple allele?

Explain the size of atoms, and define *atomic radius*.

What are some common models of atoms?

Define *atomic number*, give the symbol that represents atomic number, and name what the atomic number is equal to for atoms with a neutral charge.

Define *atomic mass*, and give the symbol that represents atomic mass.

Give the equation for finding the atomic mass, and give the reason for why the mass of electrons is basically insignificant.

Atoms are extremely small. A hydrogen atom is about 5×10^{-8} mm in diameter. According to some estimates, five trillion hydrogen atoms could fit on the head of a pin.

Atomic radius refers to the average distance between the nucleus and the outermost electron.

Each gene is made up of only two alleles, but in some cases, there are more than two possibilities for what those two alleles might be. For example, in blood typing, there are three alleles (A, B, O), but each person has only two of them. A gene with more than two possible alleles is known as a multiple allele. A gene that can result in two or more possible forms or expressions is known as a polymorphic gene.

The atomic number of an element refers to the **number of protons** in the nucleus of an atom. It is a unique identifier.

It can be represented as Z.

Atoms with a neutral charge have an atomic number that is equal to the **number of electrons**.

Models of atoms that include the proton, nucleus, and electrons typically show the electrons very close to the nucleus and revolving around it, similar to how the Earth orbits the sun.

However, another model relates the Earth as the nucleus and its atmosphere as electrons, which is the basis of the term "**electron cloud**."

Another description is that electrons swarm around the nucleus. It should be noted that these atomic models are not to scale.

A more accurate representation would be a nucleus with a diameter of about 2 cm in a stadium. The electrons would be in the bleachers. This model is similar to the not-to-scale solar system model.

The atomic mass (A) is equal to the number of protons (Z) plus the number of neutrons (N). This can be represented by the equation $A = Z + N$.

The mass of electrons in an atom is basically insignificant because it is so small.

Atomic mass is also known as the **mass number**. The atomic mass is the *total number of protons and neutrons* in the nucleus of an atom.

It is referred to as A.

What is atomic weight?

How are isotopes represented?

Explain what makes an isotope stable, name the number of known stable isotopes, and name the stable and radioactive isotopes of carbon.

Describe radioactive isotopes, and note what can be done with the knowledge about rates of decay of isotopes.

Name where electrons orbit in the atom, and describe a few of their characteristics.

What are valence shells and valence electrons?

Isotopes are atoms of the same element that vary in their number of neutrons. Isotopes of the same element have the same number of protons and thus the same atomic number. They are denoted by the element symbol, preceded in superscript and subscript by the mass number and atomic number, respectively.

For instance, the notations for protium, deuterium, and tritium are, respectively: $^{1}_{1}H$, $^{2}_{1}H$, and $^{3}_{1}H$.

Atomic weight may sometimes be referred to as "**relative atomic mass**," but should not be confused with atomic mass.

Atomic weight is the ratio of the average mass per atom of a sample (which can include various isotopes of an element) to 1/12 of the mass of an atom of carbon-12.

Radioactive isotopes have unstable nuclei and can undergo spontaneous nuclear reactions, which results in particles or radiation being emitted.

It cannot be predicted when a specific nucleus will decay, but large groups of identical nuclei decay at predictable rates.

Knowledge about rates of decay can be used to *estimate the age of materials* that contain radioactive isotopes.

Isotopes that have not been observed to decay are **stable**, or non-radioactive, isotopes. It is not known whether some stable isotopes may have such long decay times that observing decay is not possible.

Currently, 80 elements have one or more stable isotopes. There are 256 known stable isotopes in total.

Carbon, for example, has three isotopes. Two (carbon-12 and carbon-13) are stable and one (carbon-14) is radioactive.

The outermost electron shell of an atom in its uncombined state is known as the **valence shell**. The electrons there are called **valence electrons**, and it is their number that determines bonding behavior. Atoms tend to react in a manner that will allow them to fill or empty their valence shells.

Electrons are subatomic particles that orbit the nucleus at various levels commonly referred to as **layers**, **shells**, or **clouds**. The orbiting electron or electrons account for only a fraction of the atom's mass.

They are much smaller than the nucleus, are negatively charged, and exhibit wave-like characteristics. Electrons are part of the **lepton** family of elementary particles.

Name what is involved with chemical bonds, and note the result of these chemical bonds.

Name the rule of electrons filling up the four energy levels, and name the four main energy levels of an atom.

Explain why most atoms are neutral, and explain how a molecule or atom acquires a positive or negative charge.

Explain how negative and positive ions are made, and name the result when an ionic bond is formed between ions with opposite charges.

Define *ionization*, and note what happens to gases and plasmas through ionization.

Explain how a compound is made, and explain what can be seen and determined from the interactions among the molecules of a compound.

Each of the four **energy levels** (or shells) of an atom has a maximum number of electrons they can contain.

Each level must be completely filled before electrons can be added to the **valence level**. The farther away from the nucleus an electron is, the more energy it has.

The first shell, or K-shell, can hold a maximum of 2 electrons; the second, the L-shell, can hold 8; the third, the M-shell, can hold 18; the fourth, the N-shell, can hold 32. The shells can also have **subshells**.

Chemical bonds involve a negative-positive attraction between an electron or electrons and the nucleus of an atom or nuclei of more than one atom.

The attraction keeps the atom cohesive, but also enables the formation of bonds among other atoms and molecules.

A **negative ion** is created when an atom gains electrons, while a **positive ion** is created when an atom loses electrons.

An **ionic bond** is formed between ions with opposite charges. The resulting compound is neutral.

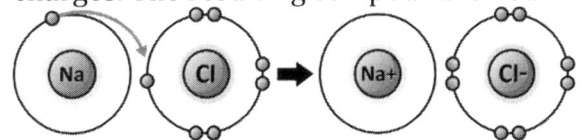

Most atoms are **neutral** since the positive charge of the protons in the nucleus is balanced by the negative charge of the surrounding electrons.

Electrons are transferred between atoms when they come into contact with each other. This creates a molecule or atom in which the number of electrons does not equal the number of protons, which gives it a positive or negative charge.

Atoms of the same element may bond together to form **molecules** or **crystalline solids**. When two or more different types of atoms bind together chemically, a **compound** is made.

The physical properties of compounds reflect the nature of the interactions among their molecules. These interactions are determined by the structure of the molecule, including the atoms they consist of and the distances and angles between them.

Ionization refers to the process by which neutral particles are ionized into charged particles. Gases and plasmas can be partially or fully ionized through ionization.

Define *chemical bonding*, and name what an atom can do with its electron when bonding with another atom.

Name the three types of chemical bonding, and explain what happens during each type.

How are cations and anions formed?

Define *ions*, and note what happens when there is a gain or a loss of electrons in an ion.

Take an atom of sodium and an atom of chlorine.
Sodium (Na): 11 electrons (including 1 electron in its outer shell).
Chlorine (Cl): 17 electrons (including 7 electrons in its outer shell).
Now, explain how sodium chloride (NaCl) is formed.

Define *covalent bonding*, and name what is produced.

Ionic bonding – When an atom gains or loses electrons it becomes negatively or positively charged, turning it into an ion. An ionic bond is a relationship between two *oppositely charged ions*.

Covalent bonding – Atoms that share electrons have what is called a covalent bond. Electrons shared equally have a *non-polar bond*, while electrons shared unequally have a *polar bond*.

Hydrogen bonding – The atom of a molecule interacts with a hydrogen atom in the same area. Hydrogen bonds can also form between two different parts of the same molecule, as in the structure of DNA and other large molecules.

A union between the electron structures of atoms is called **chemical bonding**. An atom may gain, surrender, or share its electrons with another atom it bonds with.

Atoms that lose or gain electrons are referred to as **ions**. The gain or loss of electrons will result in an ion having a positive or negative charge.

A **cation** or positive ion is formed when an atom loses one or more electrons.

An **anion** or negative ion is formed when an atom gains one or more electrons.

Covalent bonding is characterized by the sharing of one or more pairs of electrons between two atoms or between an atom and another **covalent bond**

This produces an attraction to repulsion stability that holds these molecules together.

From this, the atomic number, or number of protons, of sodium can be calculated as 11 because the number of protons equals the number of electrons in an atom.

When sodium chloride (NaCl) is formed, one electron from sodium transfers to chlorine. Ions have charges. They are written with a plus (+) or minus (−) symbol. Ions in a compound are attracted to each other because they have *opposite charges*.

$$Na\cdot + \overset{\times\times}{\underset{\times\times}{:Cl:}} \longrightarrow [Na]^+ [\overset{\times\times}{\underset{\times\times}{:Cl:}}]^-$$

electron transfer from sodium to chlorine

Life and Physical Sciences
© Mometrix Media – flashcardsecrets.com/teas
ATI TEAS Science

Name the result of an atom's tendency to share electrons with other atoms, and describe the strength for the resultant bonds of these combining atoms.

Life and Physical Sciences
© Mometrix Media – flashcardsecrets.com/teas
ATI TEAS Science

Name what items are involved most frequently with covalent bonding, and explain why nonmetals are more likely to form covalent bonds than metals.

Life and Physical Sciences
© Mometrix Media – flashcardsecrets.com/teas
ATI TEAS Science

Name when electron sharing takes place, and name two processes where covalent bonding of metals is important.

Life and Physical Sciences
© Mometrix Media – flashcardsecrets.com/teas
ATI TEAS Science

Define *electronegativity*, and explain what happens when the electronegative difference between two atoms is small, when it is large, and when there is no electronegativity.

Life and Physical Sciences
© Mometrix Media – flashcardsecrets.com/teas
ATI TEAS Science

Explain the features and formation of compounds, and name the smallest independent unit of an element or compound.

Life and Physical Sciences
© Mometrix Media – flashcardsecrets.com/teas
ATI TEAS Science

What are diatomic elements?

Covalent bonding occurs most frequently between atoms with similar **electronegativities**.

Nonmetals are more likely to form covalent bonds than metals since it is more difficult for nonmetals to liberate an electron.

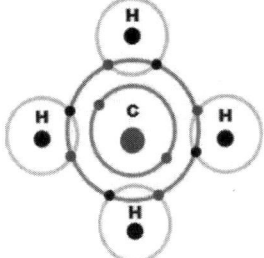

Atoms have the tendency to share electrons with each other so that all outer electron shells are filled.

The resultant bonds are always stronger than the **intermolecular hydrogen bond** and are similar in strength to ionic bonds.

Electronegativity is a measure of how capable an atom is of attracting a pair of bonding electrons. It refers to the fact that one atom exerts slightly more force in a bond than another, creating a **dipole**.

If the electronegative difference between two atoms is small, the atoms will form a **polar covalent bond**. If the difference is large, the atoms will form an **ionic bond**. When there is no electronegativity, a **pure nonpolar covalent bond** is formed.

Electron sharing takes place when one species encounters another species with similar electronegativity.

Covalent bonding of metals is important in both *process chemistry* and *industrial catalysis*.

Most elements are found somewhere in nature in single-atom form, but a few elements only exist naturally in pairs. These are called **diatomic elements**, of which some of the most common are hydrogen, nitrogen, and oxygen.

An **element** is the most basic type of matter. It has unique properties and cannot be broken down into other elements. The smallest unit of an element is the **atom**. A chemical combination of two or more types of elements is called a **compound**.

Compounds often have properties that are very different from those of their constituent elements.

The smallest independent unit of an element or compound is known as a **molecule**.

Life and Physical Sciences
© Mometrix Media – flashcardsecrets.com/teas
ATI TEAS Science

Explain how elements and compounds are represented, and give examples with water and methane.

Life and Physical Sciences
© Mometrix Media – flashcardsecrets.com/teas
ATI TEAS Science

What is a tabular arrangement of the elements that is organized by periodic law?

Life and Physical Sciences
© Mometrix Media – flashcardsecrets.com/teas
ATI TEAS Science

Note what the periodic table shows about the properties of elements, and explain the periods and groups on the table.

Life and Physical Sciences
© Mometrix Media – flashcardsecrets.com/teas
ATI TEAS Science

How are metals, metalloids, and nonmetals displayed in the periodic table of elements?

Life and Physical Sciences
© Mometrix Media – flashcardsecrets.com/teas
ATI TEAS Science

What do most periodic tables contain in each element's box?

Life and Physical Sciences
© Mometrix Media – flashcardsecrets.com/teas
ATI TEAS Science

What does the position of an element in the periodic table reveal about what kind of element that it is?

The **periodic table** is a tabular arrangement of the elements and is organized according to **periodic law**.

Elements and compounds are represented by **chemical symbols**, one or two letters, most often the first in the element name.

More than one atom of the same element in a compound is represented with a subscript number designating how many atoms of that element are present.

Water, for instance, contains two hydrogens and one oxygen. Thus, the chemical formula is H_2O. Methane contains one carbon and four hydrogens, so its formula is CH_4.

Elements are further categorized as metals, metalloids, or nonmetals. The majority of known elements are metals; there are seventeen nonmetals and eight metalloids. **Metals** are situated at the left end of the periodic table, **nonmetals** to the right and **metalloids** between the two.

The properties of the elements depend on their **atomic structure** and vary with **atomic number**. So, the table shows periodic trends of physical and chemical properties and identifies families of elements with similar properties.

In the periodic table, the elements are arranged by atomic number in horizontal rows called **periods** and vertical columns called **groups** or **families**.

The position of an element in the table reveals its group, its block, and whether it is a representative, transition, or inner transition element. Its position also shows the element as a metal, nonmetal, or metalloid.

A typical periodic table shows the elements' symbols and atomic number, the number of protons in the atomic nucleus. Some more detailed tables also list **atomic mass, electronegativity**, and other data.

Life and Physical Sciences
© Mometrix Media – flashcardsecrets.com/teas
ATI TEAS Science

What does the last digit of the group number for the representative elements and the roman numerals for the A groups reveal?

Life and Physical Sciences
© Mometrix Media – flashcardsecrets.com/teas
ATI TEAS Science

Explain what the position of the element in the table reveals about its electron configuration and how it differs in atomic size from neighbors in its period or group. Use Boron as an example.

Life and Physical Sciences
© Mometrix Media – flashcardsecrets.com/teas
ATI TEAS Science

Name the most important feature of the periodic table, and name what this feature enables with the periodic table.

Life and Physical Sciences
© Mometrix Media – flashcardsecrets.com/teas
ATI TEAS Science

Name the most important characteristic for the groups/families of elements while using the noble gases as an example, and note whether classifications rely more on groups or periods.

Life and Physical Sciences
© Mometrix Media – flashcardsecrets.com/teas
ATI TEAS Science

Define *reactivity*, and explain what reactivity depends upon.

Life and Physical Sciences
© Mometrix Media – flashcardsecrets.com/teas
ATI TEAS Science

Note what periodicity allows us to do, and explain why the elements on the right side of the periodic table are less likely to react.

The position of the element in the table reveals its **electronic configuration** and how it differs in atomic size from neighbors in its period or group. In this example, Boron has an atomic number of 5 and an atomic weight of 10.811. It is found in group 13, in which all atoms of the group have 3 valence electrons; the group's Roman numeral representation is IIIA.

For the representative elements, the last digit of the **group number** reveals the number of outer-level electrons. Roman numerals for the A groups also reveal the number of outer level electrons within the group.

Groups of elements share predictable characteristics, the most important of which is that their outer energy levels have the same configuration of electrons. For example, the highest group is group 18, the noble gases. Each element in this group has a full complement of electrons in its outer level, making the reactivity low.

Elements in periods also share some common properties, but most classifications rely more heavily on groups.

The most important feature of the table is its arrangement according to **periodicity**, or the predictable trends observable in atoms. The arrangement enables classification, organization, and prediction of important elemental properties.

Periodicity allows us to predict an element's reactivity based on its position on the periodic table.

High numbered groups on the right side of the table have a fuller complement of electrons in their outer levels, making them less likely to react. Noble gases, on the far right of the table, each have eight electrons in the outer level, with the exception of He, which has two. Because atoms tend to lose or gain electrons to reach an ideal of eight in the outer level, these elements have very low reactivity.

Reactivity refers to the tendency of a substance to engage in **chemical reactions**. If that tendency is high, the substance is said to be highly reactive, or to have **high reactivity**.

Because the basis of a chemical reaction is the transfer of electrons, reactivity depends upon the presence of uncommitted electrons which are available for transfer.

What is notable about the number of electrons within a period as you read from left to right?

What is notable about the connection of electrons to the nucleus as you read to the right of a period and as you read down a group?

Describe the role of principal energy levels with valence electrons, and note what this allows for the noble gases.

What is the location of the metals, nonmetals, and metalloids on the periodic table?

Note what metals include, and name some examples of metals.

Note what is included with nonmetals and metalloids, and name some examples of nonmetals and metalloids.

As electrons are added, their attraction to the nucleus increases, meaning that as we read to the right in a period, each atom's electrons are more densely compacted, more strongly bound to the nucleus, and less likely to be pulled away in reactions.

As we read down a group, each successive atom's outer electrons are less tightly bound to the nucleus, thus increasing their reactivity, because the principal energy levels are increasingly full as we move downward within the group.

Reading left to right within a period, each element contains one more electron than the one preceding it. (Note that H and He are in the same period, though nothing is between them and they are in different groups.)

The **metals** are located on the left side and center of the periodic table, and the nonmetals are located on the right side of the periodic table. The metalloids or semimetals form a zigzag line between the metals and nonmetals.

Principal energy levels shield the outer energy levels from nuclear attraction, allowing the valence electrons to react. For this reason, noble gases farther down the group can react under certain circumstances.

Nonmetals include the **chalcogens** such as oxygen and sulfur, the **halogens** such as fluorine and chlorine, and the **noble gases** such as helium and argon. Carbon, nitrogen, and phosphorus are also nonmetals. **Metalloids** or **semimetals** include boron, silicon, germanium, antimony, and polonium.

Metals include the alkali metals, alkaline earth metals, the transition metals, and the inner transition metals.

Some examples of **alkali metals** are lithium, sodium, and potassium. Examples of **alkaline earth metals** are beryllium, magnesium, and calcium.

Examples of **transition metals** are iron, copper, and nickel. Some examples of the **inner transition metals** are thorium, uranium, and plutonium.

Explain intensive properties, and give examples of intensive properties.

Explain extensive properties, and give examples of extensive properties.

Define *physical properties*, and name what can be included among these properties.

Define *mass*, *weight*, and *volume*, and explain a common formula for determining volume.

Define *density* and *specific gravity*, and give the formula that is used to determine density.

Explain the difference between an object's density and a material's density, and explain how an object with a very high material density may still float.

Extensive properties *do* depend on the amount of matter or quantity of the sample. Therefore, extensive properties do change if the sample size is increased or decreased. If the sample size is increased, the property increases. If the sample size is decreased, the property decreases.

Extensive properties include volume, mass, weight, energy, entropy, number of moles, and electrical charge.

Intensive properties *do not* depend on the amount of matter or quantity of the sample. This means that intensive properties will not change if the sample size is increased or decreased.

Intensive properties include color, hardness, melting point, boiling point, density, ductility, malleability, specific heat, temperature, concentration, and magnetization.

Mass is a measure of the amount of substance in an object. **Weight** is a measure of the gravitational pull of Earth on an object. **Volume** is a measure of the amount of space occupied.

There are many formulas to determine volume. For example, the volume of a cube is the length of one side cubed (a^3) and the volume of a rectangular prism is length times width times height ($l \times w \times h$). The volume of an irregular shape can be determined by how much water it displaces.

Physical properties are any property of matter that can be **observed** or **measured**. These include properties such as color, elasticity, mass, volume, and temperature.

It is important to note the difference between an *object's density* and a *material's density*. Water has a density of one gram per cubic centimeter, while steel has a density approximately eight times that.

Despite having a much higher material density, an object made of steel may still float. A hollow steel sphere, for instance, will float easily because the density of the object includes the air contained within the sphere.

Density is a measure of the amount of mass per unit volume. The formula to find density is mass divided by volume ($D=m/V$). It is expressed in terms of mass per cubic unit, such as grams per cubic centimeter (g/cm^3).

Specific gravity is a measure of the ratio of a substance's density compared to the density of water.

Define *specific heat capacity*, provide an example (using lead and magnesium) to explain how every element has its own specific heat, and give the equation for relating heat energy to specific heat capacity.

Explain the direction that heat travels, and describe what happens when two regions are at the same temperature.

Define *conduction*, and explain why heat can be transferred from one location to another by contact.

Explain what makes a property a chemical property, and use an example that involves hydrogen gas being burned in oxygen.

Name the important properties of water, and note why water is essential to life as we know it.

Explain some of the features of water regarding its liquid and solid state, and explain what it means for water to have a high specific heat.

Heat always flows from a region of higher temperature to a region of lower temperature. If two regions are at the same temperature, there is a **thermal equilibrium** between them and there will be no **net heat transfer** between them.

Specific heat capacity, also known as **specific heat**, is the *heat capacity per unit mass*.

Every element and compound has its own specific heat. For example, it takes different amounts of heat energy to raise the temperature of the same amounts of magnesium and lead by one degree.

The equation for relating heat energy to specific heat capacity is $Q = mc\Delta T$, where m represents the mass of the object, and c represents its specific heat capacity.

If a chemical change must be carried out in order to observe and measure a property, then the property is a **chemical property**.

For example, when hydrogen gas is burned in oxygen, it forms water. This is a chemical property of hydrogen because after burning, a different chemical substance – water – is all that remains. The hydrogen cannot be recovered from the water by means of a physical change such as freezing or boiling.

Conduction is a form of heat transfer that requires contact.

Since heat is a measure of kinetic energy, most commonly vibration, at the atomic level, it may be transferred from one location to another or one object to another by contact.

Water is a liquid at room temperature. In its solid state, water floats. (Most substances are heavier in their solid forms.)

The high specific heat of water means it resists the breaking of its hydrogen bonds and resists heat and motion, which is why it has a relatively high boiling point and high vaporization point. It also resists temperature change.

The important properties of water (H_2O) are *high polarity, hydrogen bonding, cohesiveness, adhesiveness, high specific heat, high latent heat, and high heat of vaporization*.

It is **essential to life** as we know it, as water is one of the main if not the main constituent of many living things.

Define *cohesive*, *adhesive*, and *hydrophilic*, and name the kinds of substances that readily dissolve in water.

Compare hydrogen bonds to covalent and ionic bonds, and note how hydrogen bonds can form.

Explain what it means for a water molecule to be polar, and name the figure that is made when hydrogen atoms are arranged around the oxygen atom.

Name what happens to hydrogen when it bonds with oxygen, and give some characteristics of hydrogen bonds.

Name some of the important properties that hydrogen bonds give to water, and name some of the important components of hydrogen bonds.

Name the role of transport mechanisms and the two types of passive transport mechanisms, and note whether they need energy from the cell.

Hydrogen bonds are weaker than covalent and ionic bonds, and refer to the type of attraction in an **electronegative atom** such as oxygen, fluorine, or nitrogen.

Hydrogen bonds can form within a single molecule or between molecules.

Water is **cohesive**, which means it is attracted to itself. It is also **adhesive**, which means it readily attracts other molecules.

If water tends to adhere to another substance, the substance is said to be **hydrophilic**.

Because of its cohesive and adhesive properties, water makes a good solvent. Substances, particularly those with polar ions and molecules, readily dissolve in water.

Hydrogen is **oxidized** (its number of electrons is reduced) when it bonds with oxygen to form water.

Hydrogen bonds tend not only to be weak but also short-lived. They also tend to be numerous.

A water molecule is **polar**, meaning it is partially positively charged on one end (the hydrogen end) and partially negatively charged on the other (the oxygen end).

This is because the hydrogen atoms are arranged around the oxygen atom in a close tetrahedron.

Transport mechanisms allow for the movement of substances through membranes.

Passive transport mechanisms include simple and facilitated diffusion and osmosis. They do not require energy from the cell.

Hydrogen bonds give water many of its important properties, including its high specific heat and high heat of vaporization, its solvent qualities, its adhesiveness and cohesiveness, its hydrophilic qualities, and its ability to float in its solid form.

Hydrogen bonds are also an important component of *proteins, nucleic acids, and DNA.*

Define *diffusion*, and give some examples of diffusion.

Define *facilitated diffusion*, and give some examples of things that are transported by carrier proteins.

Define *osmosis*, give some examples of osmosis, and describe the control that a plant has on water supply.

Name what matter refers to, and give the traditional three states of matter.

Describe the differences in the distances and angles between molecules or atoms with the three different states of matter.

What is the fourth state of matter in the current definition?

Facilitated diffusion occurs when specific molecules are transported by a specific carrier protein. **Carrier proteins** vary in terms of size, shape, and charge.

Glucose and amino acids are examples of substances transported by carrier proteins.

Diffusion occurs when particles are transported from areas of higher concentration to areas of lower concentration. When equilibrium is reached, diffusion stops.

Examples are gas exchange (carbon dioxide and oxygen) during photosynthesis and the transport of oxygen from air to blood and from blood to tissue.

Matter refers to substances that *have mass and occupy space* (or volume). The traditional definition of matter describes it as having three states: solid, liquid, and gas.

Osmosis is the diffusion of water through a semi-permeable membrane from an area of lower solute concentration to one of higher solute concentration. Examples of osmosis include the absorption of water by plant roots and the alimentary canal.

Plants lose and gain water through osmosis. A plant cell that swells because of water retention is said to be **turgid**.

The current definition of matter describes it as having four states. The fourth is **plasma**, which is an ionized gas that has some electrons that are described as free because they are not bound to an atom or molecule.

However, the TEAS will only be concerned with solids, liquids, and gases.

These different states are caused by differences in the distances and angles between molecules or atoms, which result in differences in the energy that binds them.

Solid structures are rigid or nearly rigid and have strong bonds.

Molecules or atoms of **liquids** move around and have weak bonds, although they are not weak enough to readily break.

Molecules or atoms of **gases** move almost independently of each other, are typically far apart, and do not form bonds.

How can solid become a liquid and how can a liquid form into a solid?

How can a liquid form into a gas?

Explain how it can be observed that water is less dense in its liquid state, and explain what the consequence would be if water behaved as other substances do when temperatures drop below the freezing point of a substance.

Explain the reason for the lower density of ice, and explain why there are empty spaces in the molecular structure of ice.

Visit *mometrix.com/academy* for related videos.
Enter video codes: 742449 and 802024

Give the name of the process where a solid is converted into a gas and the process where a gas is converted into a solid.

Define *evaporation*.

The three states of matter can be traversed by the addition or removal of **heat**.

For example, when a solid is heated to its melting point, it can begin to form a liquid. However, in order to transition from solid to liquid, additional heat must be added at the melting point to overcome the **latent heat of fusion**.

Upon further heating to its boiling point, the liquid can begin to form a gas, but again, additional heat must be added at the boiling point to overcome the **latent heat of vaporization**.

In the solid state, water is less dense than in the liquid state. This can be observed quite simply by noting that an ice cube floats at the surface of a glass of water.

Were this not the case, ice would not form on the surface of lakes and rivers in those regions of the world where the climate produces temperatures below the freezing point.

If water behaved as other substances do, lakes and rivers would freeze from the bottom up, which would be detrimental to many forms of aquatic life.

The lower density of ice occurs because of a combination of the unique structure of the water molecule and hydrogen bonding. In the case of ice, each oxygen atom is bound to four hydrogen atoms, two covalently and two by hydrogen bonds.

This forms an ordered roughly **tetrahedral** structure that prevents the molecules from getting close to each other. As such, there are empty spaces in the structure that account for the low density of ice.

Direct transitions from gas to solid and solid to gas are much less common in everyday life, but they can occur given the proper conditions. Solid to gas conversion is known as **sublimation**, while the reverse is called **deposition**.

Evaporation is the change of state in a substance from a liquid to a gaseous form at a temperature below its boiling point (the temperature at which all of the molecules in a liquid are changed to gas through vaporization).

Life and Physical Sciences
© Mometrix Media – flashcardsecrets.com/teas
ATI TEAS Science

Describe the actions of molecules at the surface of liquids and the actions of molecules in a substance that is at higher temperatures.

Life and Physical Sciences
© Mometrix Media – flashcardsecrets.com/teas
ATI TEAS Science

Explain what affects the rate of evaporation.

Life and Physical Sciences
© Mometrix Media – flashcardsecrets.com/teas
ATI TEAS Science

Define *condensation*.

Life and Physical Sciences
© Mometrix Media – flashcardsecrets.com/teas
ATI TEAS Science

Explain the results on a material's component molecules when temperatures decrease in a gas.

Life and Physical Sciences
© Mometrix Media – flashcardsecrets.com/teas
ATI TEAS Science

Explain the results of an increase in the pressure exerted on a gas.

Life and Physical Sciences
© Mometrix Media – flashcardsecrets.com/teas
ATI TEAS Science

What is the role of condensation in the hydrologic cycle?

The rate of evaporation is higher when more of the surface area of a liquid is exposed (as in a large water body, such as an ocean).

The amount of moisture already in the air also affects the rate of evaporation—if there is a significant amount of water vapor in the air around a liquid, some evaporated molecules will return to the liquid.

The speed of the evaporation process is also decreased by increased **atmospheric pressure**.

Some of the molecules at the surface of a liquid always maintain enough **heat energy** to escape the cohesive forces exerted on them by neighboring molecules.

At higher temperatures, the molecules in a substance move more rapidly, increasing their number with enough energy to break out of the liquid form.

When temperatures decrease in a gas, such as water vapor, the material's component molecules move more slowly.

The decreased motion of the molecules enables **intermolecular cohesive forces** to pull the molecules closer together and, in water, establish hydrogen bonds.

Condensation is the phase change in a substance from a gaseous to liquid form; it is the opposite of evaporation or vaporization.

In the **hydrologic cycle**, this process is initiated when warm air containing water vapor rises and then cools. This occurs due to convection in the air, meteorological fronts, or lifting over high land formations.

Condensation can also be caused by an increase in the pressure exerted on a gas, which results in a decrease in the substance's volume (it reduces the distance between particles).

Life and Physical Sciences

Name how the rates of chemical reactions are determined and what influences them.

Life and Physical Sciences

Name the role of catalysts and inhibitors in the chemical reactions, and name the actions of some types of reactions (e.g., releasing energy, transferring electrons, or chemical bonds being broken down).

Life and Physical Sciences

What controls processes such as the formation of ozone and greenhouse gases in the atmosphere?

Life and Physical Sciences

Explain how a chemical equation is set up, and name some of the basic parts of chemical equations.

Life and Physical Sciences

Review the following equation for the formation of water $2H_{2(g)} + O_{2(g)} \rightarrow 2H_2O_{(l)}$, and explain the meaning of each symbol, superscript, and subscript in the equation.

Life and Physical Sciences

Give a definition for unbalanced chemical equation, and note how one can know if an equation is unbalanced.

Catalysts accelerate chemical reactions, while **inhibitors** decrease reaction rates.

Some types of reactions release energy in the form of heat and light. Some types of reactions involve the transfer of either electrons or hydrogen ions between reacting ions, molecules, or atoms. In other reactions, chemical bonds are broken down by heat or light to form **reactive radicals** with electrons that will readily form new bonds.

Chemical reactions measured in human time can take place quickly or slowly. They can take a fraction of a second or billions of years.

The **rates** of chemical reactions are determined by how frequently reacting atoms and molecules interact. Rates are also influenced by the temperature and various properties (such as shape) of the reacting materials.

Chemical equations describe chemical reactions.

The **reactants** are on the left side before the arrow and the **products** are on the right side after the arrow. The arrow indicates the **reaction** or change.

The **coefficient**, or stoichiometric coefficient, is the number before the element, and indicates the ratio of reactants to products in terms of moles.

Processes such as the formation of ozone and greenhouse gases in the atmosphere and the burning and processing of fossil fuels are controlled by radical reactions.

An **unbalanced equation** is one that does not follow the **law of conservation of mass**.

If an equation is unbalanced, the numbers of atoms indicated by the stoichiometric coefficients on each side of the arrow will not be equal.

The 2 preceding hydrogen and water is the coefficient, which means there are 2 moles of hydrogen and 2 of water. There is 1 mole of oxygen, which does not have to be indicated with the number 1.

In parentheses, g stands for gas, l stands for liquid, s stands for solid, and aq stands for aqueous solution (a substance dissolved in water). **Charges** are shown in superscript for individual ions, but not for ionic compounds.

Polyatomic ions are separated by parentheses so the ion will not be confused with the number of ions.

Life and Physical Sciences
© Mometrix Media – flashcardsecrets.com/teas
ATI TEAS Science

Explain the steps for determining whether an equation is unbalanced, and balance the following equation: $H_2 + O_2 \rightarrow H_2O$

Life and Physical Sciences
© Mometrix Media – flashcardsecrets.com/teas
ATI TEAS Science

What does the Law of Conservation of Mass state?

Life and Physical Sciences
© Mometrix Media – flashcardsecrets.com/teas
ATI TEAS Science

Name what the Law of Conservation of Mass means for the total mass of material, and explain what this allows for making predictions on molecules.

Life and Physical Sciences
© Mometrix Media – flashcardsecrets.com/teas
ATI TEAS Science

Determine whether the following is balanced or unbalanced:
Two hydrogen molecules combine with one oxygen molecule to form water.

Life and Physical Sciences
© Mometrix Media – flashcardsecrets.com/teas
ATI TEAS Science

Name how chemical reactions normally occur, and explain how reactions and reactivity depend on the octet rule.

Life and Physical Sciences
© Mometrix Media – flashcardsecrets.com/teas
ATI TEAS Science

Name the general changes that come from a reaction and what results in being generated from a reaction. (Use the reaction of oxygen with methane to provide an example.)

The **Law of Conservation of Mass** in a chemical reaction is commonly stated as follows:
In a chemical reaction, matter is neither created nor destroyed.

This is a balanced chemical equation because the number of each type of atom is the same on both sides of the arrow. It has to balance because the reaction obeys the Law of Conservation of Mass.

The changes in a reaction may be in **composition** or **configuration** of a compound or substance, and result in one or more products being generated which were not present in isolation before the reaction occurred.

For instance, when oxygen reacts with methane (CH_4), water and carbon dioxide are the products; one set of substances ($CH_4 + O$) was transformed into a new set of substances ($CO_2 + H_2O$).

Start by writing the formulas for each species in the reaction. Count the atoms on each side and determine if the number is equal. **Coefficients** must be whole numbers. Fractional amounts, such as half a molecule, are not possible. Equations can be **balanced** by multiplying the coefficients by a constant that will produce the smallest possible whole number coefficient.

The balanced equation is $2H_2 + O_2 \rightarrow 2H_2O$, which indicates that it takes two moles of hydrogen and one of oxygen to produce two moles of water.

What this means is that there will always be the same **total mass** of material after a reaction as before.

This allows for predicting how molecules will combine by balanced equations in which the number of each type of atom is the same on either side of the equation.

Chemical reactions normally occur when electrons are transferred from one atom or molecule to another.

Reactions and reactivity depend on the **octet rule**, which describes the tendency of atoms to gain or lose electrons until their outer energy levels contain eight.

Life and Physical Sciences
© Mometrix Media – flashcardsecrets.com/teas
ATI TEAS Science

What is dependent on a reaction?

Life and Physical Sciences
© Mometrix Media – flashcardsecrets.com/teas
ATI TEAS Science

What are some reaction conditions or environmental factors that are important components in reactions?

Life and Physical Sciences
© Mometrix Media – flashcardsecrets.com/teas
ATI TEAS Science

Explain combination reactions, and show equation examples of the following combination reactions:
1) Burning Hydrogen in air to produce water
2) Water and Sulfur Trioxide react to form Sulfuric Acid

Life and Physical Sciences
© Mometrix Media – flashcardsecrets.com/teas
ATI TEAS Science

Define *decomposition reactions*, note the difference for the byproducts of these reactions, and note the difference between decomposition reactions and combination reactions.

Life and Physical Sciences
© Mometrix Media – flashcardsecrets.com/teas
ATI TEAS Science

Describe the role of heat in decomposition and thermal decomposition reactions, name the type of reaction that is the decomposition of water into hydrogen and oxygen gas, and give the chemical equation as well.

Life and Physical Sciences
© Mometrix Media – flashcardsecrets.com/teas
ATI TEAS Science

Name the categories of separation processes, name the properties affected when separated products differ from the original mixture, and list the types of separation processes.

Reaction conditions, or environmental factors, are also important components in reactions. These include conditions such as temperature, pressure, concentration, whether the reaction occurs in solution, the type of solution, and presence or absence of catalysts.

Reactions depend on the presence of a **reactant**, or substance undergoing change, a **reagent**, or partner in the reaction less transformed than the reactant (such as a catalyst), and **products**, or the final result of the reaction.

Decomposition (or *desynthesis, decombination, deconstruction,* or *analysis*) reactions are considered chemical reactions whereby a single compound breaks down into component parts or simpler compounds (A → B + C).

When a compound or substance separates into these simpler substances, the **byproducts** are often substances that are different from the original.

Decomposition can be viewed as the *opposite* of combination reactions.

Combination reactions: In a combination reaction, two or more reactants combine to make one product. This can be seen in the equation A + B → AB. These reactions are also known as synthesis or addition reactions.

An example is burning hydrogen in air to produce water. The equation is $2H_2$ (g) + O_2 (g) → $2H_2O$ (l).

Another example is when water and sulfur trioxide react to form sulfuric acid. The equation is H_2O + SO_3 → H_2SO_4.

Separation processes can be **mechanical** or **chemical**, and usually involve reorganizing a mixture of substances without changing their chemical nature.

The separated products may differ from the original mixture in terms of chemical or physical properties.

Types of separation processes include **filtration, crystallization, distillation,** and **chromatography**.

Most decomposition reactions are **endothermic**. Heat needs to be added for the chemical reaction to occur. **Thermal decomposition** is caused by heat.

Electrolytic decomposition is due to electricity. An example of this type of reaction is the decomposition of water into hydrogen and oxygen gas. The equation is $2H_2O$ → $2H_2$ + O_2.

Define *single substitution reactions*, and name the two categories of single substitution reactions.

Visit *mometrix.com/academy* for a related video.
Enter video code: 442975

Explain what happens when a piece of copper (Cu) is placed into a solution of silver nitrate ($AgNO_3$), and give the chemical equation for this example.

Define *double displacement reactions,* and give an example of silver nitrate and sodium chloride forming two different products with the chemical equation as well.

Name what happens to the oxidation state in a double replacement reaction.

Name the roles that acids and bases play in acid/base reactions, and describe the results of these types of reactions.

Name one method of determining whether a reaction is an oxidation/reduction or a metathesis reaction.

When a piece of copper (Cu) is placed into a solution of silver nitrate (AgNO$_3$), the solution turns blue. The copper appears to be replaced with a silvery-white material. The equation is 2AgNO$_3$ + Cu → Cu(NO$_3$)$_2$ + 2Ag.

When this reaction takes place, the copper dissolves and the silver in the silver nitrate solution precipitates (becomes a solid), thus resulting in copper nitrate and silver. Copper and silver have switched places in the nitrate.

Single substitution, displacement, or replacement reactions occur when one reactant is displaced by another to form the final product (A + BC → B + AC). Single substitution reactions can be **cationic** or **anionic**.

Double replacement reactions are **metathesis reactions**. In a double replacement reaction, the chemical reactants exchange ions but the oxidation state stays the same. One of the indicators of this is the formation of a **solid precipitate**.

Double displacement, double replacement, substitution, metathesis, or ion exchange reactions occur when ions or bonds are exchanged by two compounds to form different compounds (AC + BD → AD + BC).

An example of this is that silver nitrate and sodium chloride form two different products (silver chloride and sodium nitrate) when they react. The formula for this reaction is AgNO$_3$ + NaCl → AgCl + NaNO$_3$.

One method of determining whether a reaction is an oxidation/reduction or a metathesis reaction is that the oxidation number of atoms does not change during a metathesis reaction.

In acid/base reactions, an **acid** is a compound that can donate a proton, while a **base** is a compound that can accept a proton.

In these types of reactions, the acid and base react to form a salt and water. When the proton is donated, the base becomes **water** and the remaining ions form a **salt**.

Define *combustion*, and name some types of combustion.

Note what determines the compounds formed by a combustion reaction, and name the resulting compounds of air and burning wood.

Define *exothermic*, and name other forms that can be released from exothermic energy.

Define *catalysts*, and name what the mass of the catalyst should be at the beginning of the reaction and at the end of the reaction.

Define *activation energy*, and name the role of activation energy and catalysts in chemical reactions.

What are the catalysts in the following: the catalyst in the decomposition of hydrogen peroxide, the catalyst in the manufacture of ammonia using the Haber process, and the catalyst in the nitration of benzene?

Fuels and oxidants determine the **compounds** formed by a combustion reaction. For example, when rocket fuel consisting of hydrogen and oxygen combusts, it results in the formation of water vapor.

When air and wood burn, resulting compounds include nitrogen, unburned carbon, and carbon compounds.

Combustion, or burning, is a sequence of chemical reactions involving **fuel** and an **oxidant** that produces heat and sometimes light.

There are many types of combustion, such as rapid, slow, complete, turbulent, microgravity, and incomplete.

Catalysts, substances that help *change the rate of reaction* without changing their form, can increase reaction rate by decreasing the number of steps it takes to form products.

The **mass** of the catalyst should be the same at the beginning of the reaction as it is at the end.

Combustion is an **exothermic** process, meaning it releases energy. Exothermic energy is commonly released as heat, but can take other forms, such as light, electricity, or sound.

Examples of catalysts in reactions are manganese oxide (MnO_2) in the decomposition of hydrogen peroxide, iron in the manufacture of ammonia using the Haber process, and concentrate of sulfuric acid in the nitration of benzene.

The **activation energy** is the minimum amount required to get a reaction started.

Activation energy causes particles to collide with sufficient energy to start the reaction.

A **catalyst** enables more particles to react, which lowers the activation energy.

Explain the potential of hydrogen, and connect the level of pH with the concentration of H⁺.

Name the pH level of neutral pH and the range of pH for acids and bases, and give examples of common bases and common acids.

Explain the role of a pH indicator, and explain what it means for it to be halochromic.

Name the type of solution where basic chemicals are found, give some common traits of bases, and name the word that is used to describe bases.

Name the types of ions that acids and bases yield, and name the models that can be used to describe acids and then be inverted and used to describe bases.

Why are some nonmetal oxides (e.g., Na_2O) classified as bases?

Pure water has a **neutral pH**, which is 7.

Anything with a pH lower than pure water (<7) is considered **acidic**. Anything with a pH higher than pure water (>7) is a **base**.

Drain cleaner, soap, baking soda, ammonia, egg whites, and sea water are common bases.

Urine, stomach acid, citric acid, vinegar, hydrochloric acid, and battery acid are acids.

The **potential of hydrogen** (pH) is a measurement of the *concentration of hydrogen ions* in a substance in terms of the number of moles of H^+ per liter of solution.

All substances fall between 0 and 14 on the pH scale.

A lower pH indicates a higher H^+ concentration, while a higher pH indicates a lower H^+ concentration.

Basic chemicals are usually in aqueous solution and have the following traits: a bitter taste; a soapy or slippery texture to the touch; the capacity to restore the blue color of litmus paper which had previously been turned red by an acid; the ability to produce salts in reaction with acids.

The word **alkaline** is used to describe bases.

A **pH indicator** is a substance that acts as a detector of hydrogen or hydronium ions. It is **halochromic**, meaning it changes color to indicate that hydrogen or hydronium ions have been detected.

Some **nonmetal oxides** (such as Na_2O) are classified as bases even though they do not contain hydroxides in their molecular form.

However, these substances easily produce hydroxide ions when reacted with water, which is why they are classified as bases.

While acids yield **hydrogen ions** (H^+) when dissolved in solution, bases yield **hydroxide ions** (OH^-); the same models used to describe acids can be inverted and used to describe bases— Arrhenius, Brønsted-Lowry, and Lewis.

Name some significant properties of acids that are not readily observable, and name what characterizes carboxylic acids.

Name some properties of acids that are easy to observe without any experimental apparatus, and name whether most inorganic acids being easily soluble in water and having high boiling points are properties that are more or less easily observed.

From what are the characteristic properties of acids and bases derived?

Name what the strength of an acid or base is a reflection of, and give an example of this if all of the atoms in an acid ionize and when only a few of the atoms in an acid ionize.

Name another way to think of the strength of an acid or a base, and explain why highly reactive acids and bases are strong.

Name some properties of salts, and name some common salts.

Some other properties of acids are easy to observe without any experimental apparatus. These properties include the following:
- They have a sour taste
- They change the color of litmus paper to red
- They produce gaseous H_2 in reaction with some metals
- They produce salt precipitates in reaction with bases

Other properties, while no more complex, are less easily observed. For instance, most inorganic acids are easily soluble in water and have high boiling points.

The most significant property of an acid is not readily observable and is what gives acids their unique behaviors: the **ionization of H atoms**, or their tendency to dissociate from their parent molecules and take on an electrical charge.

Carboxylic acids are also characterized by ionization, but of the O atoms.

The strength of an acid or base is a reflection of the degree to which its atoms ionize in solution.

For example, if all of the atoms in an acid ionize, the acid is said to be **strong**. When only a few of the atoms ionize, the acid is **weak**.

Acetic acid ($HC_2H_3O_2$) is a weak acid because only its O_2 atoms ionize in solution.

The characteristic properties of acids and bases derive from the tendency of atoms to ionize by donating or accepting charged particles.

Some properties of **salts** are that they are formed from acid base reactions, are ionic compounds consisting of metallic and nonmetallic ions, dissociate in water, and are comprised of tightly bonded ions.

Some common salts are sodium chloride (NaCl), sodium bisulfate, potassium dichromate ($K_2Cr_2O_7$), and calcium chloride ($CaCl_2$).

Another way to think of the strength of an acid or base is to consider its **reactivity**

Highly reactive acids and bases are strong because they tend to form and break bonds quickly and most of their atoms ionize in the process.

Life and Physical Sciences
© Mometrix Media – flashcardsecrets.com/teas
ATI TEAS Science

Name more common salts, and name some of their uses.

Scientific Reasoning
© Mometrix Media – flashcardsecrets.com/teas
ATI TEAS Science

Name the preferred system for taking measurements, and explain why a universal standard for measurements is necessary.

Scientific Reasoning
© Mometrix Media – flashcardsecrets.com/teas
ATI TEAS Science

Name the basic units of measurement and what they measure, and name the number of units that the metric system increases or decreases.

Scientific Reasoning
© Mometrix Media – flashcardsecrets.com/teas
ATI TEAS Science

Finish the following: meters in a dekameter, liters in a dekaliter, and grams in a dekagram, and name what *hecto-* and *kilo-* are times the base amount.

Scientific Reasoning
© Mometrix Media – flashcardsecrets.com/teas
ATI TEAS Science

What are the prefixes that indicate a fraction of the base unit?

Scientific Reasoning
© Mometrix Media – flashcardsecrets.com/teas
ATI TEAS Science

Name some of the fractions of seconds that SI uses to measure time.

Using the **metric system** is generally accepted as the preferred method for taking measurements.

Having a universal standard allows individuals to interpret measurements more easily, regardless of where they are located.

Calcium chloride is used as a drying agent, and may be used to absorb moisture when freezing mixtures.

Potassium nitrate (KNO_3) is used to make fertilizer and in the manufacture of explosives.

Sodium nitrate ($NaNO_3$) is also used in the making of fertilizer.

Baking soda (sodium bicarbonate) is a salt, as are Epsom salts [magnesium sulfate ($MgSO_4$)]. Salt and water can react to form a base and an acid. This is called a **hydrolysis reaction**.

The prefix and the base unit combined are used to indicate an amount.

For example, deka is 10 times the base unit. A dekameter is 10 meters; a dekaliter is 10 liters; and a dekagram is 10 grams.

The prefix hecto refers to 100 times the base amount; kilo is 1,000 times the base amount.

The basic units of measurement are: the **meter**, which measures length; the **liter**, which measures volume; and the **gram**, which measures mass.

The metric system starts with a **base unit** and increases or decreases in units of 10.

SI uses the **second** (s) to measure time. Fractions of seconds are usually measured in metric terms using prefixes such as millisecond (1/1,000 of a second) or nanosecond (1/1,000,000,000 of a second).

The prefixes that indicate a fraction of the base unit are deci, which is 1/10 of the base unit; centi, which is 1/100 of the base unit; and milli, which is 1/1000 of the base unit.

Scientific Reasoning
© Mometrix Media – flashcardsecrets.com/teas
ATI TEAS Science

Name how time is measured when the increments of time are larger than a second, and explain the meaning of a swimmer's time being described as 7:32.67

Scientific Reasoning
© Mometrix Media – flashcardsecrets.com/teas
ATI TEAS Science

Name the SI base units that are used to measure the following: electric current, thermodynamic temperature, luminous intensity, amount of a substance at a molecular level, length, and mass.

Scientific Reasoning
© Mometrix Media – flashcardsecrets.com/teas
ATI TEAS Science

Name the prefixes of multiples for the following: 10^1, 10^2, 10^3, 10^6, 10^9, and 10^{12}.

Scientific Reasoning
© Mometrix Media – flashcardsecrets.com/teas
ATI TEAS Science

Name the prefixes of subdivisions for the following: 10^{-1}, 10^{-2}, 10^{-3}, 10^{-6}, 10^{-9}, and 10^{-12}.

Scientific Reasoning
© Mometrix Media – flashcardsecrets.com/teas
ATI TEAS Science

Name the rule for capitalizing the abbreviation of a prefix that is greater than 10^3, and note the need for periods after abbreviating prefixes and the need for making an abbreviation plural.

Scientific Reasoning
© Mometrix Media – flashcardsecrets.com/teas
ATI TEAS Science

Name the role of graduated cylinders, name the materials that are used to make these cylinders, and compare the characteristics of those materials to glass.

Other SI base units are the **ampere** (A) (used to measure electric current), the **kelvin** (K) (used to measure thermodynamic temperature), the **candela** (cd) (used to measure luminous intensity), and the **mole** (mol) (used to measure the amount of a substance at a molecular level).

Meter (m) is used to measure length and **kilogram** (kg) is used to measure mass.

Increments of time larger than a second are measured in minutes and hours, which are multiples of 60 and 24.

An example of this is a swimmer's time in the 800-meter freestyle being described as 7:32.67, meaning 7 minutes, 32 seconds, and 67 one-hundredths of a second.

One second is equal to 1/60 of a minute, 1/3,600 of an hour, and 1/86,400 of a day.

The prefixes for subdivisions are as follows:
deci (d), 10^{-1}
centi (c), 10^{-2}
milli (m), 10^{-3}
micro (µ), 10^{-6}
nano (n), 10^{-9}
pico (p), 10^{-12}

The prefixes for multiples are as follows:
deka (da), 10^1 (deka is the American spelling, but deca is also used)
hecto (h), 10^2
kilo (k), 10^3
mega (M), 10^6
giga (G), 10^9
tera (T), 10^{12}

Graduated cylinders are used for precise measurements and are considered more accurate than flasks or beakers.

They are made of either **polypropylene** (which is shatter-resistant and resistant to chemicals but cannot be heated) or **polymethylpentene** (which is known for its clarity).

They are lighter to ship and less fragile than glass.

The rule of thumb is that prefixes greater than 10^3 are capitalized when abbreviating.

Abbreviations do not need a period after them.

A decimeter (dm) is a tenth of a meter, a deciliter (dL) is a tenth of a liter, and a decigram (dg) is a tenth of a gram. Pluralization is understood.

For example, when referring to 5 mL of water, no "s" needs to be added to the abbreviation.

Scientific Reasoning
© Mometrix Media – flashcardsecrets.com/teas
ATI TEAS Science

Explain how to read a graduated cylinder, and note how to avoid breaking a graduated cylinder if one is tipped over.

Scientific Reasoning
© Mometrix Media – flashcardsecrets.com/teas
ATI TEAS Science

Explain the role of burettes, compare the appearance of a burette to a graduated cylinder, and name the equipment that can fill a burette.

Scientific Reasoning
© Mometrix Media – flashcardsecrets.com/teas
ATI TEAS Science

Name the two types of flasks commonly used in lab settings, and name what can be used for mixing, transporting, and reacting but are not for accurate measurements.

Scientific Reasoning
© Mometrix Media – flashcardsecrets.com/teas
ATI TEAS Science

Explain the use of a pipette, describe how to read a pipette measurement, and name some types of pipettes.

Scientific Reasoning
© Mometrix Media – flashcardsecrets.com/teas
ATI TEAS Science

Name the three types of balances that measure mass and force, and rank the accuracy of each balance from most to least accurate.

Scientific Reasoning
© Mometrix Media – flashcardsecrets.com/teas
ATI TEAS Science

Explain the parts and the role of the triple-beam balance.

A **burette**, or buret, is a piece of lab glassware used to accurately dispense liquid.

It looks similar to a narrow graduated cylinder, but includes a stopcock and tip. It may be filled with a funnel or pipette.

A **pipette** can be used to accurately measure small amounts of liquid. Liquid is drawn into the pipette through the bulb and a finger is then quickly placed at the top of the container.

The liquid measurement is read exactly at the **meniscus**. Liquid can be released from the pipette by lifting the finger.

There are also plastic disposal pipettes. A **repipette** is a hand-operated pump that dispenses solutions.

One part of a triple-beam balance is the **plate**, which is where the item to be weighed is placed.

There are also three **beams** that have hatch marks indicating amounts and hold the weights that rest in the notches.

The front beam measures weights between 0 and 10 grams, the middle beam measures weights in 100 gram increments, and the far beam measures weights in 10 gram increments.

The sum of the weight of each beam is the total weight of the object.

To read a graduated cylinder, it should be placed on a flat surface and read at eye level. The surface of a liquid in a graduated cylinder forms a lens-shaped curve. The measurement should be taken from the bottom of the curve.

A ring may be placed at the top of tall, narrow cylinders to help avoid breakage if they are tipped over.

Two types of flasks commonly used in lab settings are **Erlenmeyer flasks** and **volumetric flasks**, which can also be used to accurately measure liquids.

Erlenmeyer flasks and **beakers** can be used for mixing, transporting, and reacting, but are not appropriate for accurate measurements.

Unlike laboratory glassware that measures volume, **balances** such as triple-beam balances, spring balances, and electronic balances measure **mass** and **force**.

An **electronic balance** is the most accurate, followed by a **triple-beam balance** and then a **spring balance**.

Scientific Reasoning
© Mometrix Media – flashcardsecrets.com/teas
ATI TEAS Science

Name the parts of a triple beam balance that calibrate the equipment, and indicate that the object and counterweights are in balance. Also, note the accuracy of analytical balances.

Scientific Reasoning
© Mometrix Media – flashcardsecrets.com/teas
ATI TEAS Science

What is needed for a valid experiment?

Scientific Reasoning
© Mometrix Media – flashcardsecrets.com/teas
ATI TEAS Science

Explain what a researcher should know in advance of an experiment, and note what a researcher needs to ensure for data that is collected.

Scientific Reasoning
© Mometrix Media – flashcardsecrets.com/teas
ATI TEAS Science

How can a researcher validate the measurement system?

Scientific Reasoning
© Mometrix Media – flashcardsecrets.com/teas
ATI TEAS Science

Name one thing that scientists must not allow in their data collection, and explain why hypothesizing is an important skill for scientists.

Scientific Reasoning
© Mometrix Media – flashcardsecrets.com/teas
ATI TEAS Science

Name the three skills that the data-analysis process requires, and describe the importance of how gathered data should be arranged.

A valid experiment must be measurable. **Data tables** should be formed, and meticulous, detailed data should be collected for every trial.

A triple beam balance also includes a **set screw** to calibrate the equipment and a mark indicating the object and counterweights are in balance.

Analytical balances are accurate to within 0.0001 g.

The researcher should validate the measurement system by performing **practice tests** and making sure that all of the equipment is correctly **calibrated** and periodically retesting the procedure and equipment to ensure that all data being collected are still valid.

First, the researcher must determine exactly what data are needed and why those data are needed.

The researcher should know in advance what will be done with those data at the end of the experimental research.

The data should be *repeatable, reproducible, and accurate*. The researcher should be sure that the procedure for data collection will be reliable and consistent.

The **data-analysis process** requires the twin skills of ordering and categorizing. A skill that may be integrated with the previous two is comparing.

Gathered data must be arranged in such a way that it is readable and readily shows the key results, and scientists should be able to **compare** their own results with other published results.

Perhaps the most important skill in science is that of **observation**.

Scientists must be able to take accurate data from their experimental setup or from nature without allowing bias to alter the results.

Another important skill is **hypothesizing**. Scientists must be able to combine their knowledge of theory and of other experimental results to logically determine what should occur in their own tests.

Scientific Reasoning
© Mometrix Media – flashcardsecrets.com/teas
ATI TEAS Science

Explain the importance of scientists applying their knowledge of theory, and explain the importance of scientists communicating their results and their conclusions.

Scientific Reasoning
© Mometrix Media – flashcardsecrets.com/teas
ATI TEAS Science

Define *hypotheses*, and name the things that can be the basis for hypotheses.

Scientific Reasoning
© Mometrix Media – flashcardsecrets.com/teas
ATI TEAS Science

Define *assumptions*, and explain why assumptions are necessary.

Scientific Reasoning
© Mometrix Media – flashcardsecrets.com/teas
ATI TEAS Science

Define *scientific models*, explain why some models can be discarded, and explain a model's usefulness.

Scientific Reasoning
© Mometrix Media – flashcardsecrets.com/teas
ATI TEAS Science

What is the difference between scientific laws and theories?

Scientific Reasoning
© Mometrix Media – flashcardsecrets.com/teas
ATI TEAS Science

Explain the difference between a cause and an effect, and name some terms that are used to signal causes, and name terms that can be used to signal effects.

Hypotheses are educated guesses about what is likely to occur, and are made to provide a starting point from which to begin design of the experiment.

They may be based on results of previously observed experiments or knowledge of theory, and follow logically forth from these.

They must also be able to **infer**, or draw logical conclusions, from their results. They must be able to **apply** their knowledge of theory and results to create logical experimental designs and determine cases of special behavior.

Lastly, scientists must be able to **communicate** their results and their conclusions. The greatest scientific progress is made when scientists are able to review and test one another's work and offer advice or suggestions.

Scientific models are mathematical statements that describe a physical behavior. Models are only as good as our knowledge of the actual system.

Often models will be discarded when new discoveries are made that show the model to be inaccurate.

While a model can never perfectly represent an actual system, they are useful for simplifying a system to allow for better understanding of its behavior.

Assumptions are statements that are taken to be fact without proof for the purpose of performing a given experiment. They may be entirely true, or they may be true only for a given set of conditions under which the experiment will be conducted.

Assumptions are necessary to simplify experiments; indeed, many experiments would be impossible without them.

A **cause** is an act or event that makes something happen, and an **effect** is the thing that happens as a result of the cause.

A cause-and-effect relationship is not always explicit, but there are some terms in English that signal causes, such as *since*, *because*, and *due to*. Terms that signal effects include *consequently, therefore, this lead(s) to*.

Scientific laws are statements of natural behavior that have stood the test of time and have been found to produce accurate and repeatable results in all testing.

A **theory** is a statement of behavior that consolidates all current observations. Theories are similar to laws in that they describe natural behavior, but are more recently developed and are more susceptible to being proved wrong. Theories may eventually become laws if they stand up to scrutiny and testing.

Scientific Reasoning
© Mometrix Media – flashcardsecrets.com/teas
ATI TEAS Science

Give an example of how a single cause can have multiple effects.

Scientific Reasoning
© Mometrix Media – flashcardsecrets.com/teas
ATI TEAS Science

Give an example of how a single effect can have multiple causes.

Scientific Reasoning
© Mometrix Media – flashcardsecrets.com/teas
ATI TEAS Science

Give an example of how an effect can in turn be the cause of another effect.

Scientific Reasoning
© Mometrix Media – flashcardsecrets.com/teas
ATI TEAS Science

Why is it important to know which unit of measurement is needed to record the length or width and the weight of an object?

Scientific Reasoning
© Mometrix Media – flashcardsecrets.com/teas
ATI TEAS Science

Name the accepted units when measuring a patient's height versus measuring a patient's vein, and name the accepted way to measure a patient's weight versus measuring the weight of a human heart.

Scientific Reasoning
© Mometrix Media – flashcardsecrets.com/teas
ATI TEAS Science

Name the accepted units when measuring a patient's lifespan, and name the accepted way to measure the number of breaths that a patient takes.

A *single* effect can have *multiple* causes.

Single effect: Alan has a fever.

Multiple causes: An unexpected cold front came through the area, and Alan forgot to take his multi-vitamin to avoid being sick.

A *single* cause can have *multiple* effects.

Single cause: Because you left your homework on the table, your dog engulfs the assignment.

Multiple effects: As a result, you receive a failing grade; your parents do not allow you to visit your friends; you miss out on the new movie and holding the hand of a potential significant other.

From the largest objects in outer space to the smallest pieces of the human body, there are objects that can come in many different sizes and shapes. Many of those objects need to be measured in different ways.

So, it is important to know which **unit of measurement** is needed to record the length or width and the weight of an object.

An *effect* can in turn be the cause of *another effect*, in what is known as a **cause-and-effect chain**.

As a result of her disdain for procrastination, Lynn prepared for her exam. This led to her passing her test with high marks. Hence, her resume was accepted and her application was approved.

The same idea for scale holds true with time as well. When measuring the lifespan of a patient, the accepted measure is given in days, months, or years.

However, when measuring the number of breaths that a patient takes, the accepted measure is given in terms of minutes (e.g., breaths per minute).

An example is taking the measurements of a patient. When measuring the total height of a patient or finding the length of an extremity, the accepted measure is given in meters. However, when one is asked for the diameter of a vein, the accepted measure is given in millimeters.

Another example would be measuring the weight of a patient which would be given in kilograms, while the measurement of a human heart would be given in grams.

Scientific Reasoning
ATI TEAS Science

Define *scientific method*, and explain why the first step of the scientific method is essential.

Scientific Reasoning
ATI TEAS Science

Once a problem has been defined, what is the next step in the scientific method?

Scientific Reasoning
ATI TEAS Science

Name the next step of the scientific method once a hypothesis has been formed, and name the key to making the best possible use of this step.

Scientific Reasoning
ATI TEAS Science

Discuss the difference between quantitative measurements and qualitative measurements.

Scientific Reasoning
ATI TEAS Science

What are the necessary steps after drawing conclusions about the results of the experiment?

Scientific Reasoning
ATI TEAS Science

Why must every stage of an experiment be carefully planned?

The **scientific method** of inquiry is a general method by which ideas are tested and either confirmed or refuted by experimentation.

The first step in the scientific method is **formulating the problem** that is to be addressed. It is essential to define clearly the limits of what is to be observed, since that allows for a more focused analysis.

Once the problem has been defined, it is necessary to form a **hypothesis**. This educated guess should be a possible solution to the problem that was formulated in the first step.

The next step is to test that hypothesis by **experimentation**. This often requires the scientist to design a complete experiment.

The key to making the best possible use of an experiment is observation.

Designing relevant experiments that allow for meaningful results is not a simple task. Every stage of the experiment must be carefully planned to ensure that the right data can be safely and accurately taken.

Observations may be **quantitative**, that is, when a numeric measurement is taken, or they may be **qualitative**, that is, when something is evaluated based on feeling or preference. This measurement data will then be examined to find trends or patterns that are present.

From these trends, the scientist will draw **conclusions** or make **generalizations** about the results, intended to predict future results.

If these conclusions support the original hypothesis, the experiment is complete and the scientist will publish his conclusions to allow others to test them by repeating the experiment.

If they do not support the hypothesis, the results should then be used to develop a new hypothesis, which can then be verified by a new or redesigned experiment.

Scientific Reasoning
ATI TEAS Science

Explain the reason that experiments should be controlled, and name an example of a control in a drug trial.

Scientific Reasoning
ATI TEAS Science

Name what should be kept in mind when designing an experiment, and name what the data can be reviewed for especially if there are data points that are orders of magnitude from the expected value.

Scientific Reasoning
ATI TEAS Science

Name some ways for data to be analyzed once all the data have been gathered.

Scientific Reasoning
ATI TEAS Science

Name the one variable that is not kept exactly the same during an experiment, and name what the control group represents in a set of data.

Scientific Reasoning
ATI TEAS Science

What is the difference between positive controls and negative controls?

Scientific Reasoning
ATI TEAS Science

Will an experiment have more valid conclusions if they come from an experiment that is well controlled?

In addition to proper control, it is important that the experiment be designed with **data collection** in mind. For instance, if the quantity to be measured is temperature, there must be a temperature device such as a thermocouple integrated into the experimental setup.

While the data are being collected, they should periodically be checked for obvious errors.

If there are data points that are orders of magnitude from the expected value, then it might be a good idea to make sure that no experimental errors are being made, either in data collection or condition control.

A valid experiment must be carefully **controlled**. All variables except the one being tested must be carefully maintained. This means that all conditions must be kept exactly the same except for the independent variable.

Additionally, a set of data is usually needed for a **control group**. The control group represents the "normal" state or condition of the variable being manipulated.

The better an experiment is controlled, the more valid the conclusions from that experiment will be.

A researcher is more likely to draw a valid conclusion if all variables other than the one being manipulated are being controlled.

Ideally, an experiment should be **controlled** so that all of the conditions except the ones being manipulated are held **constant**.

This helps to ensure that the results are not skewed by unintended consequences of shifting conditions.

A good example of this is a placebo group in a drug trial. All other conditions are the same, but that group is not given the medication.

Once all the data have been gathered, they must be **analyzed**. The way in which this should be done depends on the type of data and the type of trends observed.

It may be useful to fit curves to the data to determine if the trends follow a common mathematical form.

It may also be necessary to perform a statistical analysis of the results to determine what effects are significant. Data should be clearly presented.

Controls can be negative or positive. **Positive controls** are the variables that the researcher expects to have an effect on the outcome of the experiment. A positive control group can be used to verify that an experiment is set up properly.

Negative control groups are typically thought of as placebos. A negative control group should verify that a variable has no effect on the outcome of the experiment.

Explain the difference between independent and dependent variables.

Visit *mometrix.com/academy* for related videos.
Enter video codes: 627181 and 565738

Name the independent variable, the dependent variable, and the constants for testing the effect of temperature on the solubility of a solute.

Every experiment has several **variables**; however, only one variable should be purposely changed and tested. This variable is the **manipulated** or **independent variable**. As this variable is manipulated or changed, another variable, called the **responding** or **dependent variable**, is observed and recorded.

All other variables in the experiment must be carefully controlled and are usually referred to as **constants**.

For example, when testing the effect of temperature on solubility of a solute, the independent variable is the temperature, and the dependent variable is the solubility.

All other factors in the experiment such as pressure, amount of stirring, type of solvent, type of solute, and particle size of the solute are the constants.